Manual of Ultrasound in Obstetrics and Gynaecology

W0036882

"To strive, to seek, to find.........
.... and not to yield".

Manual of Ultrasound in Obstetrics and Gynaecology

Kakoli Ghosh Dastidar

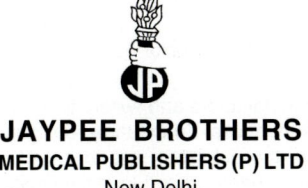

JAYPEE BROTHERS
MEDICAL PUBLISHERS (P) LTD
New Delhi

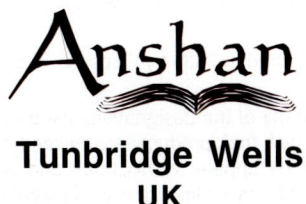

Tunbridge Wells
UK

First published in the UK by

Anshan Ltd
in 2005
6 Newlands Road
Tunbridge Wells
Kent TN4 9AT, UK

Tel/Fax: +44 (0)1892 557767
E-mail: info@anshan.co.uk
www.anshan.co.uk

Copyright © 2003 by (author)

The right of (editor) to be identified as the editor of this work has been asserted in accordance with the Copyright, Designs and Patents act 1988.

ISBN 1 904798 373

British Library Cataloguing in Publication Data
A catalogue record for this book is available from the British Library

All rights reserved. No part of this publication may be reproduced, stored in a retrieval system, or transmitted in any form or by any means, electronic, mechanical, photocopying, recording and/or otherwise without the prior written permission of the publishers. This book may not be lent, resold, hired out or otherwise disposed of by way of trade in any form, binding or cover other than that in which it is published, without the prior consent of the publishers.

Printed in India by Gopsons Papers Ltd., A-14, Sector 60,Noida

Many of the designations used by manufacturers and sellers to distinguish their products are claimed as trademarks. Where those designations appear in this book and where the publisher was aware of a trademark claim, the designations have been printed in initial capital letters.

to
my inspiration ——
Dr Sudarsan Ghosh Dastidar
and my family

Foreword

Since the introduction by Ian McDonald in 1958 ultrasound has improved dramatically and is now the most important noninvasive technique in obstetrics and gynaecology. Ultrasound is used in many diagnostic and therapeutic procedures. This book discusses very elegantly various important aspects of ultrasound in obstetrics and gynaecology, including basic physics and safety, Doppler ultrasonography, prenatal diagnosis of congenital abnormalities and the application of ultrasound in infertility. Furthermore a chapter deals on new developments like 3-Dimensional ultrasound.

This book contains important new data and clear illustrations and is therefore highly recommended for gynaecologists, residents, medical students and ultrasonographers.

Jim Van Eyck MD, PhD
Department of Perinatal Medicine
Isala Clinics Location Sophia
Zwolle—The Netherlands

Preface

I have been involved in ultrasound for gynaecological and obstetric diagnostic, therapeutic purposes since 1984. In the process, I realized the dearth of training facility in our curriculum and non-availability of readily available reading material here.

This is my initial attempt for present students; and might still leave scope for improvement, but to quote *Albert Einstein* "*A person who never made a mistake never tried anything new*". I hope this book is of benefit to their learning process.

Kakoli Ghosh Dastidar

Acknowledgements

Dr Sudarsan Ghosh Dastidar, MD for valuable guidance.

Sri Pratap Kumar Chatterjee for typing the manuscript.

Contents

Chapter 1

Basic Physics of Diagnostic Ultrasound

WHAT IS DIAGNOSTIC ULTRASOUND?

Sound, as a mode of explorative studies was first developed by Professor Langevin for the First World War to fight the U-Boat menace. In a similar technique ultrasound or sound of high frequency that is beyond audible range, was used later for diagnostic purposes in medical science. It is produced electronically by converse piezoelectric effect, a property exhibited by some elements in nature called piezoelectric crystals. Piezoelectric effect was first described by Madam Curie. But now, the transducers or ultrasound producing crystals are also manufactured artificially. Like audible sound, ultrasound waves are also mechanical-pressure waves and need a medium for propagation.

The world of present day diagnostic ultrasonography was essentially a black and white one with various shades of grey between them until recently. Recent developments in vascular flow studies by Colour Doppler has added a lot of colour to this already exciting technology.

The perfection of diagnostic superiority in real time studies lies in the correct appreciation of the various shades of black colour and their respective interpretation by an experienced sonologist.

Terminology and principles that govern the passage of diagnostic ultrasound waves through tissues:

Ultrasound is sound whose frequency is beyond the audible range. They are mechanical pressure waves.

Frequency of ultrasound is given as number of cycles of waves passing a point per unit time (second). The higher the frequency, lesser is the tissue penetration. The speed at which ultrasound waves pass through the medium is called **acoustic velocity (C)** which is given by

$$C = \lambda F$$

Acoustic velocity C = Acoustic wave length × Frequency, and its value for different media are given in Table 1.1.

Table 1.1

Air	330 mt/sec
Water	1480 mt/sec
Fat	1450 mt/sec
Blood	1570 mt/sec
Kidney	1560 mt/sec
Soft tissue (average)	1540 mt/sec
Liver	1550 mt/sec
Muscle	1580 mt/sec
Bone	4080 mt/sec

Acoustic waves may be longitudinal or transverse during a study. Longitudinal waves have direction of particle motion parallel to wave velocity. Transverse waves have direction of particle motion perpendicular to wave velocity. For this reason only longitudinal waves can propagate in soft tissues of body. In a wave form of transmission, the wave length is equal to repetition distance in space for a single frequency wave.

Acoustic intensity (I) is the energy propagating through a unit area in the medium normal to the direction of propagation per unit time and is given as I = mill watt/sec.

Acoustic impedance (Z) is the obstructive capacity of the particular tissue, through which the high frequency sound is being sent, towards passage of ultrasound waves through itself. It is equal to the product of tissue density and acoustic velocity and is dependant on tissue character (density P). It is extremely important in predicting magnitude of reflected echoes at tissue interface which forms the backbone for formation of sonographic picture.

$$Z = PC$$

Acoustic impedance = Tissue density (gm/cm^3) × Acoustic velocity (cm/sec.)

Technique for measurement of distance of anatomy or pathology within the tissue is done using the time taken for pulsed sound wave to travel from the source to tissue interface (which acts as a sound reflector) and back to the echo receiver.

Using the acoustic velocity of the medium, the depth or distance is calculated using the formula.

$$R = \frac{1}{2} \, CT$$

Distance = *½ Acoustic velocity × time from source to reflector and back.*

Chapter 2

How to Focus?

Unlike other diagnostic procedures, ultrasound study needs the presence of an expert—either during the process or the expert must visualize a live recording to come to a correct diagnosis. Still photographs or films are inadequate alone to serve the purpose.

It is essential for the operator to focus the incident sound beam in the proper plane, through proper acoustic window for optimum information.

For pelvic studies done abdominally, an optimally full urinary bladder is mandatory. It helps in two ways —

1. It rises to become an abdomino-pelvic structure thus pulling the uterus, fallopian tubes and ovaries along with it.
2. It acts as an acoustic window to study the posteriorly placed organs. About 2-3 glasses of water (400-500 ml) drunk 2 hours prior to scan is sufficient.

Focussing

1. Hold transducer firmly.
2. At the onset, locate a mark on the house of transducer, given by the manufacturers/ company to signify longitudinal axis.
3. Place thumb on that mark.
4. Expose the lower abdomen, adequately (many a study has been incomplete due to faulty exposure) up to pubic hairline. Apply an even layer of coupling gel on this area with a sponge.

5. Place transducer in the midline in longitudinal axis little above the pubic hairline and give sufficient downward pressure.

6. If the bladder is optimally full the uterus comes intoview. This is the uterus in longitudinal axis.

   At times the uterus may be slightly deviated on the right or left of midline. In such as case, the transducer might have to be angled towards the right or left of midline.

7. After the longitudinal study is completed, the transducer is turned through 90^0. This will give a transverse section through the structures to be studied.

Here, let us assume the pelvic structures to be the furniture in a darkened room whose doors and windows are all locked and we are trying to look at them through a hole in the wall with a help of a beam of light of a hand held torch. In such case we would turn the beam through an arc to look at the furniture inside. To look at an object on the left the torch would have to be held in a right to left direction and the beam would pass through structures on the left of midline. Similarly, for right sided observation the beam would have to be passed from the left to the right.

So, once the transducer is turned to let the beam travel transversely rolling motion of the operator's wrist allows the modulation to rotate its incident beam for study of structure.

It is advisable to avoid:

a. Over fullness of urinary bladder—which prevents proper study especially for ovarian folliculometry, study of internal os, cervical canal and placenta praevia.

b. Too thick layer of coupling gel.

c. Leaving the transducer smeared with gel after a study.

At present pelvic study is done only by vaginal route. For transvaginal study the endocavitory transducer is covered with a fresh condom, for hygienic insertion, better picture clarity, to prevent cross infection amongst patients, before every study and cleaned with a soft cloth afterwards. Coupling gel is placed within the condom not on it. Operator must wear sterile gloves.

Chapter 3

Role of Pelvic Vaginal Sonography for Patient Evaluation and Ovulation Monitoring

PELVIC SONOGRAPHY FOR BASIC ASSESSMENT

Uterus

- Size
- Echocharacter of myometrium
- Length of cervix
- Condition of cervical canal
- Health of vaginal portion of cervix
- Diameter of external os (incompetent os is better evaluated in pregnancy state).

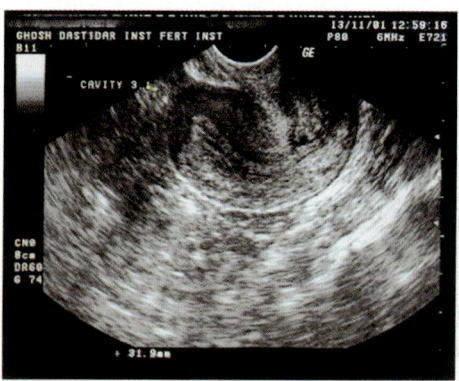

FIGURE 3.1: Normal uterus—
Anteverted, anteflexed

Endometrium

- Morphology, growth of endometrium, vascularity alteration
- Thickness.

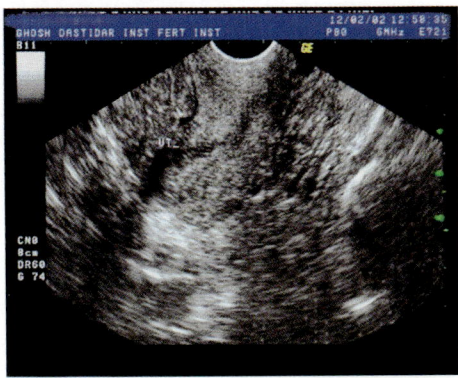

FIGURE 3.2: Retroverted small uterus

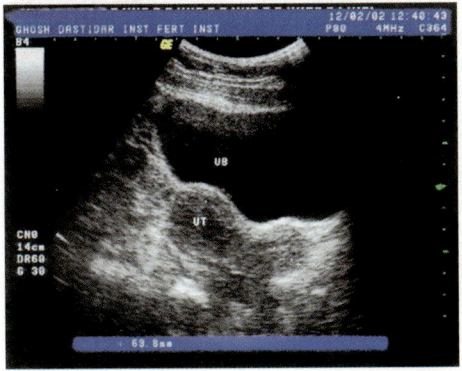

FIGURE 3.3: Uterus on abdominal ultrasound

Ovaries

- Position
- Size
- Internal echopattern of ovaries.

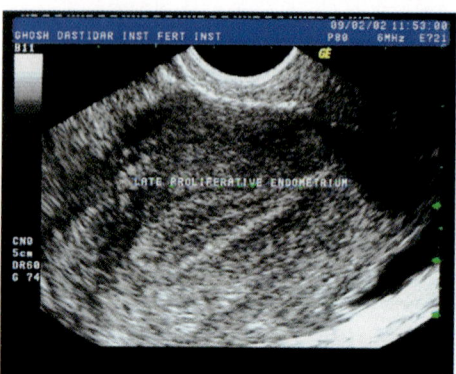

FIGURE 3.4: Late proliferative endometrium

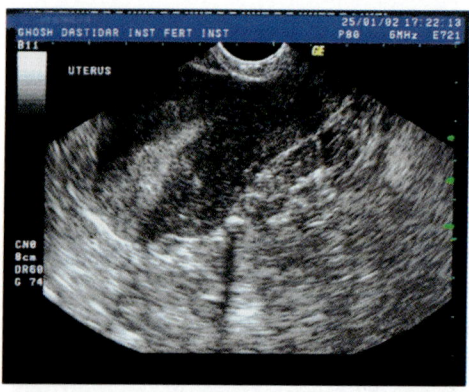

FIGURE 3.5: Adenomyotic uterus, distorted cavity, hyperechoic endometrium

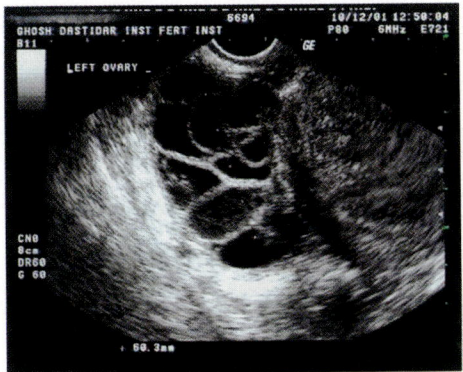

FIGURE 3.6: Multiple follicles—
Stimulated cycle

PATHOLOGY OF UTERUS, CERVIX, OVARY, FALLOPIAN TUBE STUDIED BY ULTRASOUND

- Fibroleiomyoma of uterine body or cervix.
- Adenomyosis.
- Hyperplasia, polyp, inflammation of endometrium.
- Erosion, chronic ulceration, Nabothian cyst formation of cervix.
- Ovarian masses—cystic, solid and masses of mixed echocharacter including serous cyst, mucinous—cystadenoma, papillary cystadenocarcinoma, endometrioma, mature teratoma, etc.
- Tubal pathologies like salpingitis, hydrosalpinx, fimbrial cysts or masses (normal fallopian tubes are usually not seen by routine sonography).

- Intra-pelvic adhesions both omental and local.
- Uterine scars.
- Lymph node enlargements.

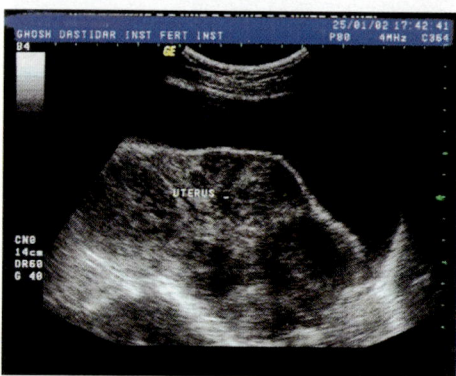

FIGURE 3.7: Multiple fibroleiomyomas
with distorted cavity

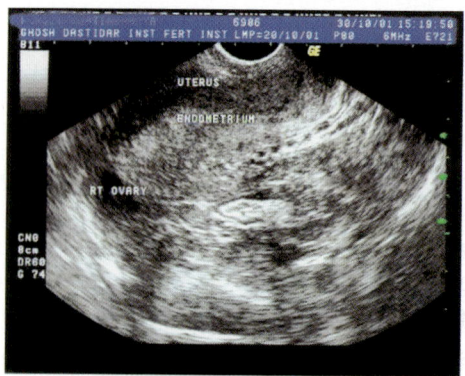

FIGURE 3.8: Adenomyosis, adherent ovary
with pelvic adhesion

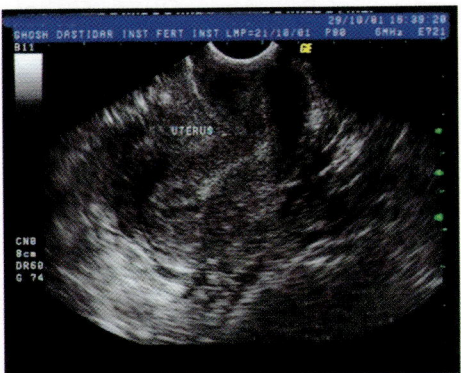

FIGURE 3.9: Inflamed endometrium

THRUST AREA—INFERTILITY

- Detects ovulatory status by serial study from D3 of cycle.
- Monitors follicular rupture and formation of corpus luteum (thereby ruling out anovulation and LUF syndrome).
- Identifies polycystic ovarian disease.
- Monitors progressive thickening and 'layering' of endometrium required for implantation.
- Measures vascular flow to ovaries, uterus and endometrium.
- Confirms implantation.
- Detects endometriosis in very early stage.
- Confirms or detects anomalies of the uterus by 3D ultrasound.

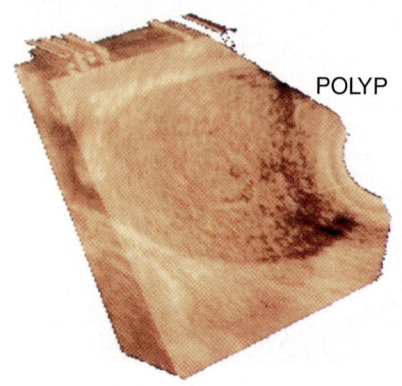

FIGURE 3.10: Polyp

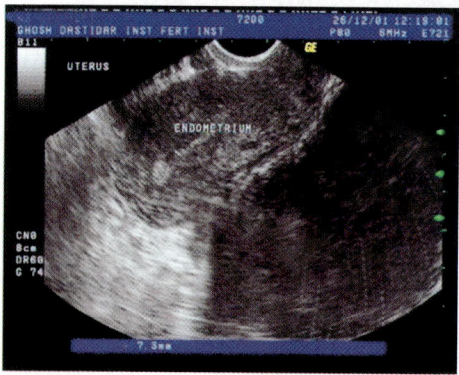

FIGURE 3.11: Patchy endometrium

Ovulatory Status by Serial Study from D3 of Cycle

Simultaneously as revolution was taking place in the reproductive laboratory around culture of pre-embryos, the ultrasound machine was going

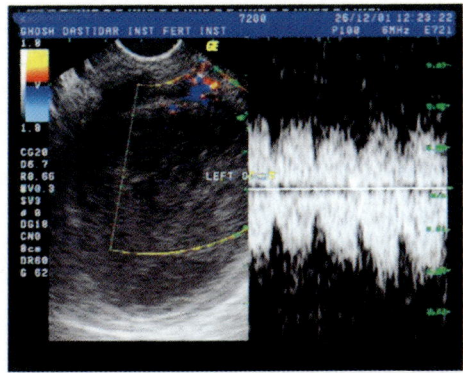

FIGURE 3.12: Endometrioma—Left ovary

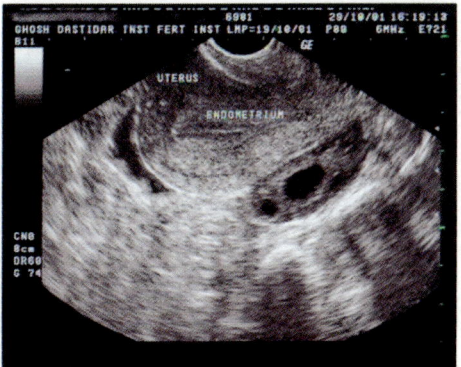

FIGURE 3.13: Pelvic inflammation

through various technical advances to get a good picture of the Pandora's box. The possibility of studying the female pelvic structures, namely uterus and ovaries, using ultrasound was first demonstrated by AK Kratochwil in 1972.

There was no looking back for the consultant treating infertile patients after the birth of Lousie Brown in U.K., Durga and Imran in Calcutta. For infertility treatment ultrasound specially trans-vaginal ultrasound became indispensable.

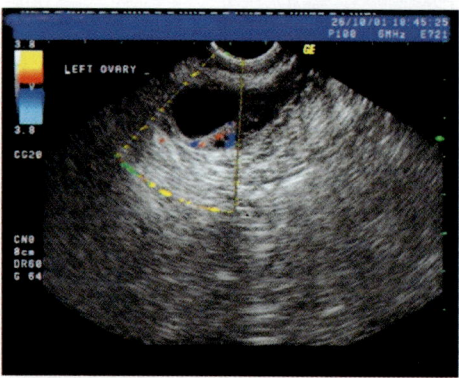

FIGURE 3.14: Follicle natural cycle

The only organ in female human body that undergoes cyclical change throughout the reproductive years are the reproductive organs. In fact, it has also been shown by Doppler ultrasound that there is even presence of Circadian rhythm in uterine artery blood flow independent of serum hormones. Such ever changing features can be monitored by serial ultrasound and patience pays in the management of infertility. So serial daily ultrasound is done from D7 of the menstrual cycle in case of unstimulated cycle to study the growth, maturation of ovarian Graffian follicle. Simultaneous study of endometrial proliferation is also done. At the present day, Doppler study is added on, which has been reported to predict normal ovulation by an alteration in the vascular flow indices. A follicle in normal cycle grows in a linear fashion and ruptures approximately around D14. However, the cycle length of every patient is different and it can rupture as late as D21 which would also be normal. Hence serial study is very important. The mature follicle has a diameter of 18-21 mm.

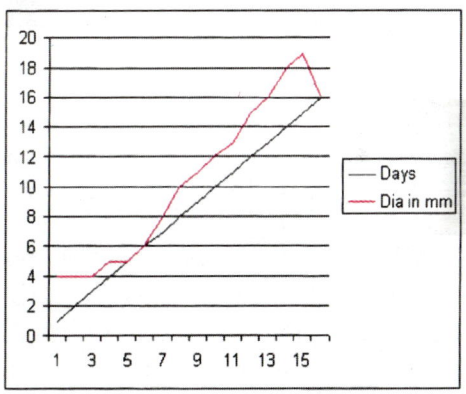

FIGURE 3.15: Growth of follicle

In oligomenorrhoeic cycles follicle might normally grow however delayed, and rupture even later or not rupture at all. Unruptured follicle that undergoes vascularisation like corpus luteum can only be detected by ultrasound and no other

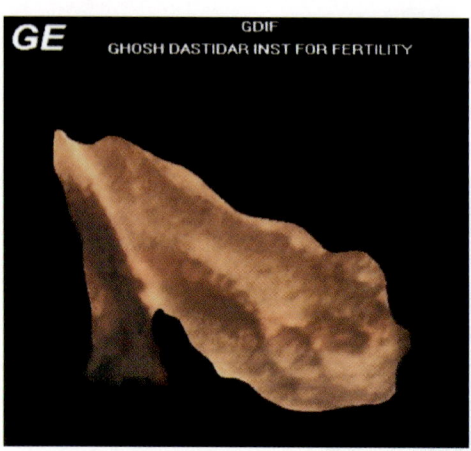

FIGURE 3.16: Ovary-3D view of follicular development

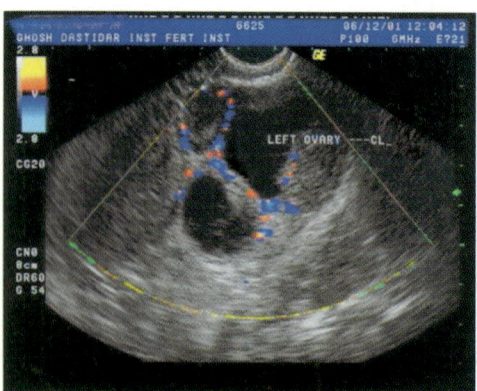

FIGURE 3.17: Healthy corpus luteum— Ring of fire on CD

biochemical test. After rupture within 24 hours the corpus luteum formation takes place and its angio-genesis gives a typical (Ring of Fire) appearance on colour Doppler study.

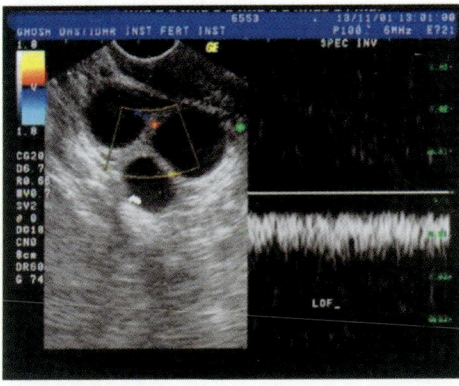

FIGURE 3.18: Anaemic corpus luteum

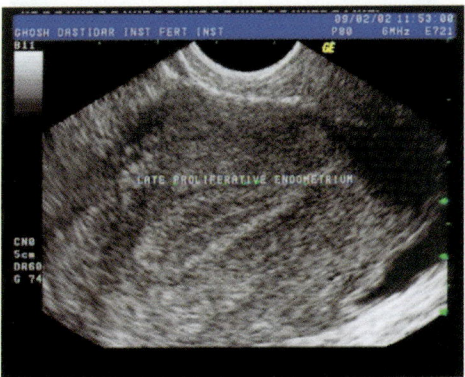

FIGURE 3.19: Endometrium

While this has been taking place the endometrium undergoes steady growth seen on ultrasound as five different layers. So much so that 2D, 3D and Doppler velocimetry studies of the endometrium has even been reported to predict successful implantation.

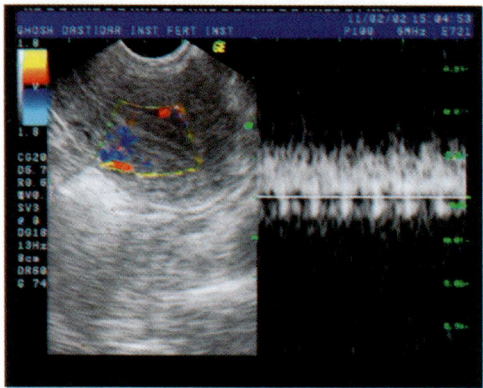

FIGURE 3.20: Radial and spiral artery

Three different varieties of endometrial echo-character have been studied and reported—(a) Isoechoic with the myometrium showing a homogeneous granular appearance, (b) Hypoechoic in comparison to myometrium, (c) Hyperechoic than the myometrium with loss of central line—resembling secretory endometrium but in the proliferative phase. The first variety has the highest implantation rate. Endometrium is measured from anterior myometrial/endometrial interphase to the posterior myometrial/endometrial interphase. A preimplantation endometrium might measure between 8 and 14 mm. Like endometrium, its spiral artery blood flow also responds to hormones throughout the cycle and grows in the proliferative phase under hormonal influence. The rupture of a follicle is confirmed by :–

a. nonvisualisation of the follicle.
b. Smaller size of follicle after a larger previous size.
c. Fluid in the POD
d. Corpus luteum on Doppler ultrasound.

Stimulated Cycle

Over the last few decades ovulation stimulatory and inducing agents have been produced by pharmaceutical companies for multifollicular growth; to be fruitful in treatment cycles. In such stimulated cycle, serial study is also necessary but it starts much earlier from D3/4 when the ovary is said to be the "quietest" and any other co-existing pathology can be ruled out.

SPECIALISED AREAS OF UTILITY

a. TVUS guided cannulation of fallopian tubes.
b. Fallopian insemination/GIFT/ ET
c. TVUS guided oocyte retrieval.
d. Cyst aspiration.

e. Management of ectopic pregnancy.
f. Multifetal reduction.
g. Fetal therapy.

Chapter 4
Doppler

DOPPLER ULTRASOUND IN GYNAECOLOGY AND OBSTETRICS

Colour Doppler studies have added to lot of colour to the grim-grey world of ultrasound. On 25th May 1852, at a meeting of the Royal Bohemian Society of Sciences in Prague, a gentleman, Christian Doppler presented a paper "On the coloured light of double stars and certain other stars of the heavens" about the red shift in light from stars. Though this has later been refuted, this effect, described by him stayed on and has been named after him. It has found a place of great prominence in noninvasive vascular studies in the human.

I have often been asked by students whether the red coloured vessels seen during a Doppler study are the arteries and the blue ones the veins. Well no!

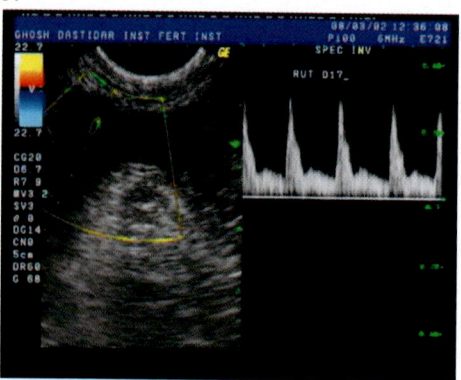

FIGURE 4.1: Doppler velocimetry of uterine artery

Let us assume that we are sitting inside a moving train which is moving at high speed and blowing its whistle. Another train is coming towards it on a track alongside at a similar speed and also blowing its whistle. When these two trains cross each other the sound volume of the whistle will have a higher frequency and we hear it louder. Similar is the case in Doppler effect.

The RBC particles in the blood vessels are moving at a speed of few cm/sec. When the ultrasound beam is directed towards these moving RBCs there will be an additive frequency shift – which looks red and if they move away from one or another the frequency change will be lower giving a blue colour on screen. For turbulent flows there are various shades of greenish-yellow between these two.

Over the last decade Doppler ultrasound has become a routine mode of study through a lot of research. The commonly measured parameters are the peak systolic flow S (in cm/sec), end-diastolic flow D (also in cm/sec), and the flow indices Pulsatility index

PI, given as S – D/ A (mean frequency shift in one cardiac cycle)

RI (resistance index) given as S-D/S.

The indices give an idea, about downstream resistance to flow or distal haemodynamics, e.g. umbilical artery flow gives idea about placental function. As they are measured in a single cardiac cycle they are virtually independent of angle of insonation. However, sample volume and wall filter adjustments are often required.

Foetal Study

After implantation, the embedding trophoblast erode maternal spiral arteries to set-up the feto-maternal circulation.

However, if during this stage improper vascularization occurs, later development of foetal growth retardation and or maternal hypertension has been reported to occur. In a large series we have reported how Doppler can detect this "Vascular Fetomaternal" crosstalk as early as 5th week of menstrual age.

In feto-placental circulation, progressive lowering of index values take place to allow continuous flow to growing organs of foetus to cause uninterrupted perfusion to vital organs. The pulsatility, i.e. the difference between maximum systolic and end diastolic flow progressively diminishes with advancing gestation. In normal pregnancies the diastolic component in the cerebral arteries is lower than in the umbilical arteries throughout pregnancy; i.e. the resistance in cerebral vessels is higher than the placental vessels and thus ratio of resistances – Cerebroplacental ratio (CPR) is greater than 1. In case of flow redistribution, as in foetal growth retardation the CPR becomes less

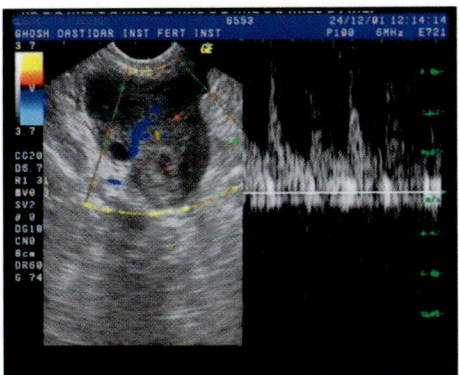

FIGURE 4.2: Ectopic trophoblast with blood flow within fallopian tube

than 1. Being a ratio of resistance in two vessels in same cardiac cycle, this value is independent of heart rate. With maternal inhalation of moist oxygen and correction of flow redistribution, CPR has been reported to become normal. The two umbilical arteries together carry approximately 40% of foetal stroke volume.

As of now the major foetal vessels being studied include the descending aorta, umbilical arteries, renal vessels, pulmonary vessels, and intracerebral vessels like internal carotid, anterior and middle cerebral arteries. Maternal arteries studied for foetal well-being are the uterine arteries, which are easy to locate at the level of internal os.

Foetal 'brain-sparing effect' by vascular flow redistribution has long been studied. Lately the 'heart sparing effect' has been reported in growth retarded foetuses. Brain sparing phenomenon has been shown to precede late deceleration of foetal heart by several weeks. However, preceding death in such cases normalization of PI and RI in cerebral vessels has also been seen. Pulsatile flow in the umbilical vein with absent or reversed end diastolic flow in the umbilical artery is the last sign of foetal asphyxia before foetal demise. This has now been reported to be accompanied by increased vascular flow in coronary arteries which has been attributed to dilatation of coronary arteries in cases of extreme foetal hypoxaemia.

In abnormal gestation such as ectopic pregnancy, when ordinary 2D ultrasound is not so efficient to detect an ectopic sac in the early stages of gestation, the typical flow—high velocity low impedance and of high diastolic flow in the adnexa is helpful for confirmation. As a concomitant feature this flow will be absent within the uterus in ectopic gestation, unless it is a rare case of heterotopic pregnancy which however has gone up after advent of various infertility management procedures and can be as high as 1 in 6000 in contrast to a previous incidence of 1 in 30,000. An ectopic pregnancy can be similar in flow pattern to a luteal cyst, cystic ovarian malignancy, tubo-ovarian abscess, pedunculated fibroid with high vascularity.

In Gynaecology

Doppler study has made it possible not only to study the pelvic anatomy but the physiology throughout the menstrual cycle by studying the various pelvic vessels and thus get information regarding vascular - functional pathophysiology. Torsion of ovarian mass results in disturbed blood flow which can be studied well.

In detection of ovarian malignancy in early stage Doppler plays an important role. Being a leading cause of gynaecologic cancer mortality, the 5 year survival rate having only increased from 36% in 1975 to 39% in 1990 it is disturbing to note that over 90% patients with stage I ovarian malignancy can be given a better prognosis with early diagnosis. Doppler has stepped in here, since other screening methods like CA 125, an antigenic determinant on a high molecular weight glycoprotein, that is recognized by the monoclonal antibody OC-125, shows a value of 35U/ml or more in majority (80%) of patients with advanced epithelial ovarian carcinoma, is elevated in only 23-50% of stage I disease. CA 125 is also elevated in other benign conditions like endometriosis, pelvic inflammatory disease, uterine fibroids, pregnancy and cirrhosis. It is also elevated in other malignant conditions of pancreas, breast, lung and endometrium and hence is not specific. But a tumour vessel of neoangiogenesis having no muscular media coat gives a typical

Doppler waveform and over 90% diagnostic accuracy has been reported by several workers in differentiating benign from malignant ovarian lesions. The PI in such lesions is less than 1.

In Infertility

Many groups have reported large series of pelvic Doppler study in normal and stimulated cycles for treatment of infertility.

Before a pelvic study, it has to be appreciated that unlike any other organ of the body, the pelvic structures involved in reproductive function undergo a cyclical hormone-related morphological and functional change which also affects the vascular function.

New vessel formation or neoangiogenesis formation takes place during follicular growth/maturation, corpus luteum formation and endometrial proliferation and layering. During follicular growth angiogenesis takes place in the thecal layer while the granulosa layer remains avascular. After ovulation thecal vessel vascularise the corpus luteum formation. Spiral arteries from the basal endometrium grow throughout the proliferative phase to supply the functional layer.

Transvaginal sonography can detect the detailed stages of the follicular growth, endometrial proliferation and measure in cm/sec, the blood flowing within them. A steady blood supply in both phases of cardiac cycles viz. systolic and diastolic is essential for growth sustenance and this is evident in normal cycles in all related vessels. It has been reported that detection of blood flow at a particular site in a growing follicle denotes healthy cumulus growth and is followed with a 70% chance of producing good (grade I or II) embryo in IVF.

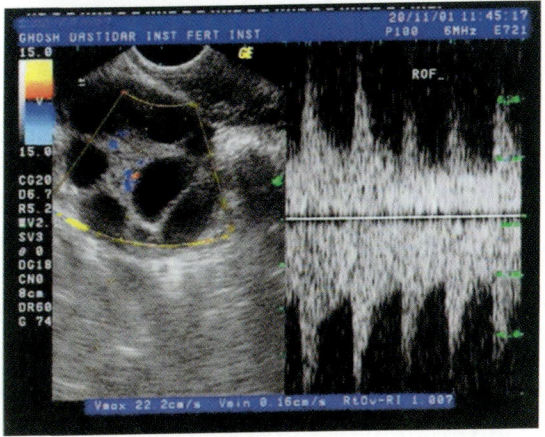

FIGURE 4.3: Blood flow in controlled ovarian stimulation

Before seeds are sown the nursery bed is prepared with care. For implantation to be successful the rose-bed, here the endometrium needs to be checked and prepared carefully. Growth in mm; measured between anterior and posterior myometrial-endometrial interphase usually is monitored throughout the follicular phase. This endometrium, divided into five zones, is capable of supporting implantation when the spiral arteries coil up along the glandular elements of the endometrium from D7. Blood flow can be measured within these vessels from D7.

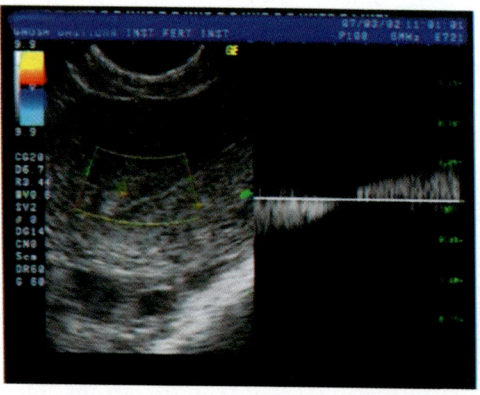

FIGURE 4.4: Pulsatile flow in endometrium

Uterine arteries and ovarian arteries are also followed throughout the cycle since high velocity flow throughout cardiac cycle with low PI is good for positive pregnancy outcome. A PI of 3 or more usually will not allow enough perfusion and thus nutrition to the embedding blastocyst. Uterine artery also shows progressively diminishing PI during luteal phase of natural cycle. In spontaneous non-conception cycles, elevated PI in mid luteal phase has been recorded to be present in women having history of unexplained recurrent pregnancy loss.

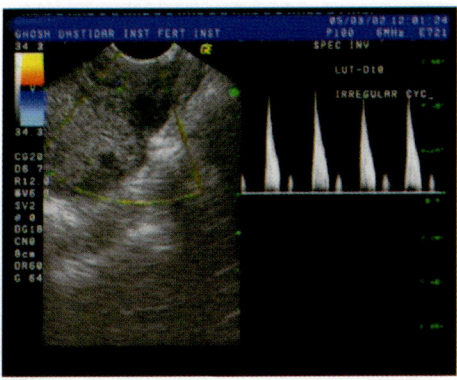

FIGURE 4.5: Circadian variation in uterine flow

Implantation vascularity has been studied very early by us and followed by, later larger series. It can be seen as early as D6/7 of implantation. Absence of such flow results in restricted growth of sac, blighted ovum and IUGR later on. Simultaneous corpus luteal blood flow which has a "Ring of Fire" appearance when healthy, rules out a nonfunctioning CL or luteal phase defect.

The velocimetric pattern is characteristic in polycystic ovarian disease, very high stromal blood flow is seen in basal studies and this is thought by some workers to be the initiating factor for higher incidence of ovarian hyperstimulation syndrome (OHSS) in such patients. However such conclusion can be reached after more detailed reports come in from workers.

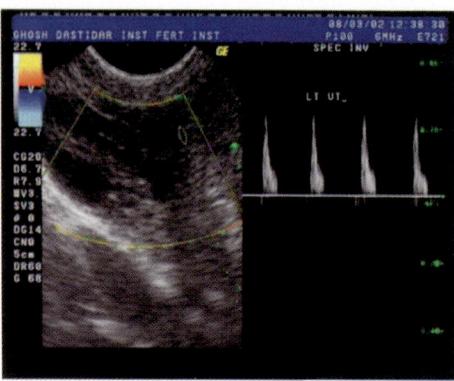

FIGURE 4.6: Poor uterine flow in women with unexplained recurrent pregnancy loss

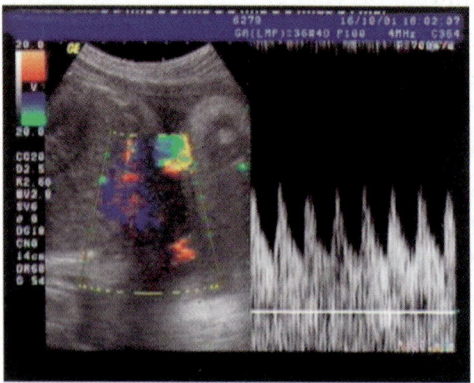

FIGURE 4.7: Umbilical artery

The blood flow of uterine, ovarian and endo-metrial vasculature in poor responders also has a characteristic pattern. In fact each vessel in the body shows a typical flow pattern.

Doppler in Pregnancy

Nearly 80% of the uterine blood supply is through the uterine arteries which reach the uterus at the level of internal os and travel along the side of the body upwards to terminate in a meso-ovarian and tubal branch. These arteries gives rise to arcuate arteries which run parallel to each other within the myometrium from these, centripetal radial arteries originate penetrating the middle third of myometrium giving rise to approximately 200 spiral arteries. The uterine artery through these branches grow in size and volume throughout pregnancy and the blood flow increases with progressive decrease in the index values. Flow parameters that do not comply to this normal status results in adverse pregnancy outcome such as intra-uterine growth retardation, pregnancy complicated by maternal hypertension and also defective placental function. High resistance uteroplacental circulation secondary to abnormal placentation can be correlated with alteration in uterine artery Doppler parameter. When studying the vessels, the ultrasound beam is made to focus in such a fashion that the angle of insonation forms 20-60 degree with the vessel and 50 Hz filter used to eliminate low frequency signals.

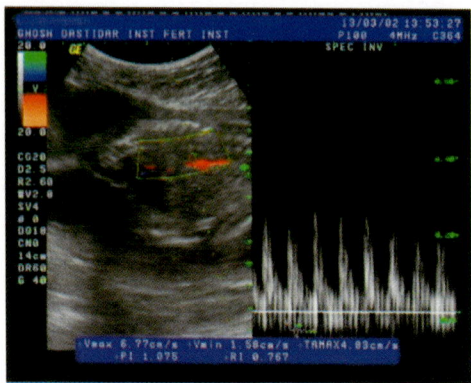

FIGURE 4.8: Foetal descending
aorta velocimetry

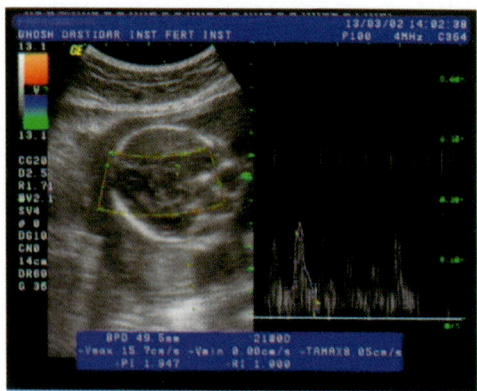

FIGURE 4.9: Measuring foetal
cerebral blood flow

Doppler to Study Effect of Vasoactive Drugs in Pregnancy

Pregnancy induced hypertension is associated with increased peripheral vascular resistance which can lead to a reduction in uteroplacental blood flow. Uteroplacental and foetal haemodynamic response to various antihypertensive drugs was controversial with divided opinion regarding advantages and disadvantages of such agents. Advent of Doppler sonography has altered the scenario such that serial studies on uterine and foetal haemodynamics and the effect of drug can be studied with high intraobserver reproducibility. No significant changes in blood flow volume in umbilical vein were observed after labetalol and prostacyclin infusion. Dihydralazine increased umbilical vein flow volume. Metoprolol, a β, adrenoreceptor antagonist elevated the resistance index in the foetal descending thoracic aorta. Atenolol, a cardio selective β blocker, shows increased uteroplacental vascular resistance, increased indices in foetal descending aorta and umbilical artery during long-term treatment. Atenolol also decreases peak velocity in foetal pulmonary trunk. Pindolol, a non-selective β blocker with vasodilatory effects did not alter resistance in any foetal artery including umbilical and middle cerebral. Nifedipine, a calcium channel blocker does not alter vascular resistance in foetal umbilical or middle cerebral arteries.

Magnesium sulfate decreases flow indices in uterine arteries and foetal cerebral arteries. In endothelial dysfunction in pre-eclampsia treatment is with nitric oxide donor substance by nitroglycerine. Such pregnancies showing foetal growth retardation and increased resistance in umbilical arteries, treated with glyceryl trinitrate shows decrease in indices of umbilical artery, signifying normalization in vascular resistance.

Doppler Studies on Obstetric, Analgesia and Anaesthesia

Maternal hypotension often accompanies regional blocks and some anaesthetic agents also have effects on maternal haemodynamics. Adrenaline added to local anaesthetics, vasopressors used for treatment of maternal hypotension and maternal postural alteration may all cause such changes in fetomaternal circulation. All of these can be accurately monitored by Doppler velocimetric studies of concerned vessels, and it has been recorded that regional blocks cause lowering of flow indices and increased blood velocity when used along with adrenaline, in uterine arteries. Indices in foetal renal and middle cerebral vessels are decreased.

After spinal anaesthesia, the flow velocity indices are increased in foetal umbilical artery.

Ephedrine and etilefrine used for treatment of maternal hypotension significantly increase vascular resistance in uterine arteries though no changes are evident in umbilical circulation, ephedrine decreases indices in foetal middle cerebral and renal arteries, enhancing the blood flow to these organs. It also has been seen to increase foetal right ventricular contractility by real time and Doppler Studies. However, the recorded minor foetal flow alterations, detected by Doppler appear to be clinically harmless, reflecting a great foetal tolerance to such situation in a normally growing foetus.

In uncompromised pregnancies the umbilical artery flow resistance does not change whereas the uterine artery flow resistance increases significantly.

Chapter 5

3-Dimensional Ultrasound in Gynaecology/ Obstetrics

Over the past years ultrasound pictures have been 2-Dimensional or flat giving the transverse and longitudinal sections. An experienced sonologist always imagined the third dimension in space, adding volume to the picture seen on the screen and created the impression mentally of the anatomical structure; as one would see it as a specimen. However, all sonologists are not experienced enough, and also at times difficulty would arise in understanding an anatomical section even by the most experienced one, particularly in understanding the tissue plane giving rise to errors in diagnosis. In particular the most difficult situations would arise in diagnosing cases of small or minor structural defect in the foetus. 3D ultrasound is invaluable in such situations. In fact 4D ultrasound

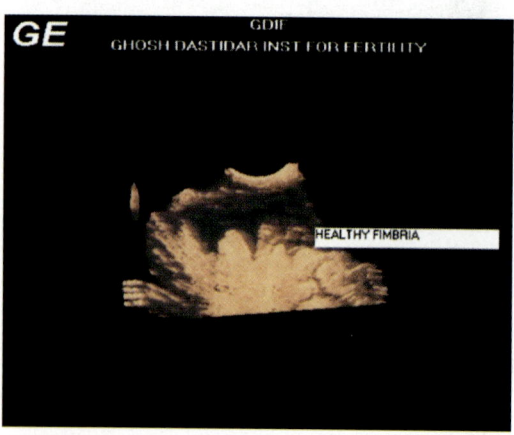

FIGURE 5.1: 3-Dimensional view—Fimbria

has also arrived which takes into account the movement of the body parts and having very high pulse repetition factor creates a near realistic picture as one would see before ones eyes.

Such a realistic picture facilitates not only the sonologist to detect pathology but makes it easier for even the consultant to understand the visualized image.

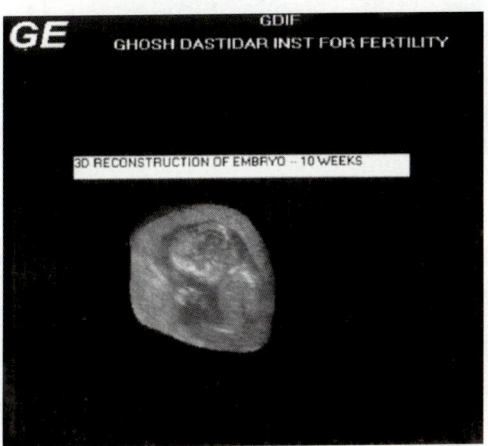

FIGURE 5.2: Foetus

It has been seen that even pregnant women can understand the picture of a baby and reports are there to suggest that such understanding creates a better fetomaternal psychological bondage. It has also been seen that previously in cases of foetal anomaly when parents were told about it, they

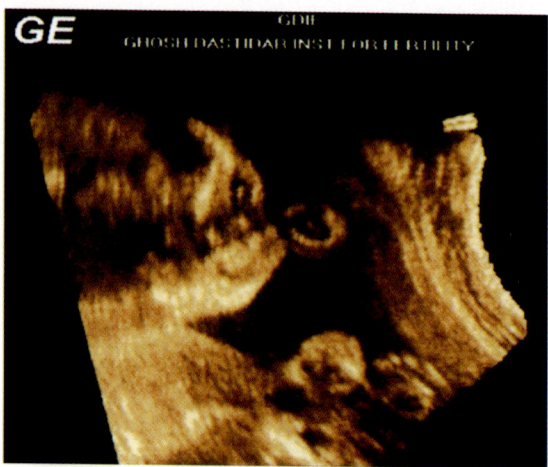

FIGURE 5.3: Facial cleft—Anomalous face

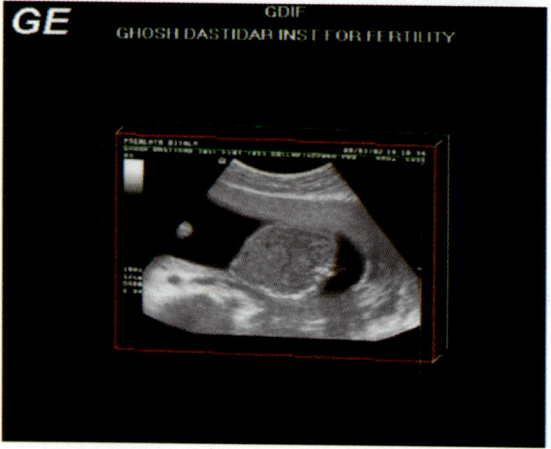

FIGURE 5.4: Lumbar meningomyelocele

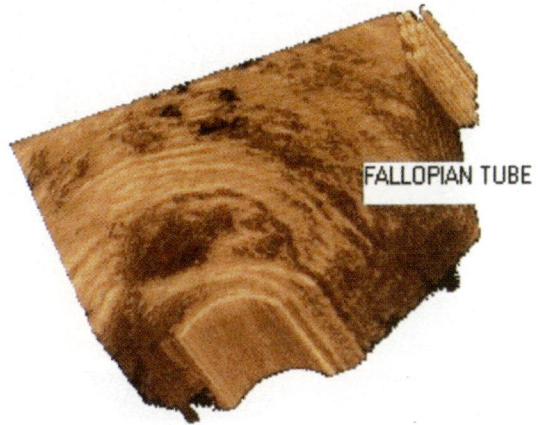

FIGURE 5.5: Fallopian tube—3D view

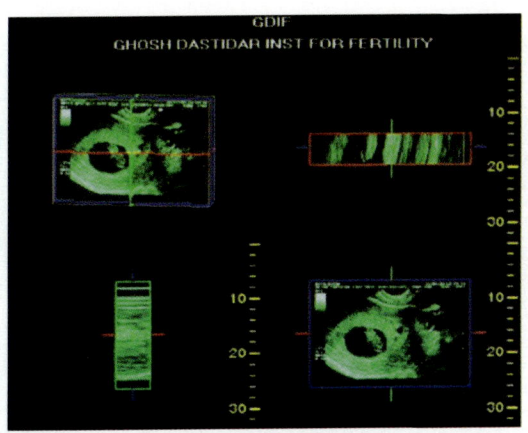

FIGURE 5.6: Multiple sections
seen on one screen

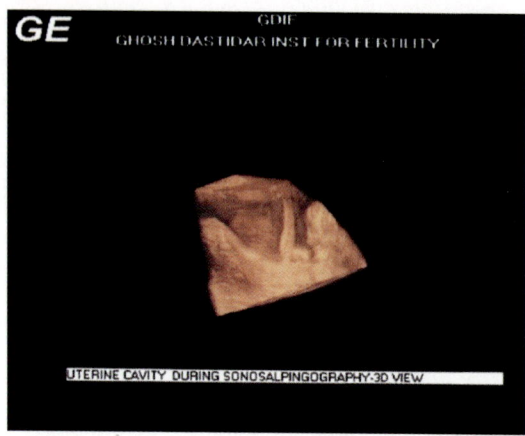

FIGURE 5.7: 3D of uterine cavity during saline infusion

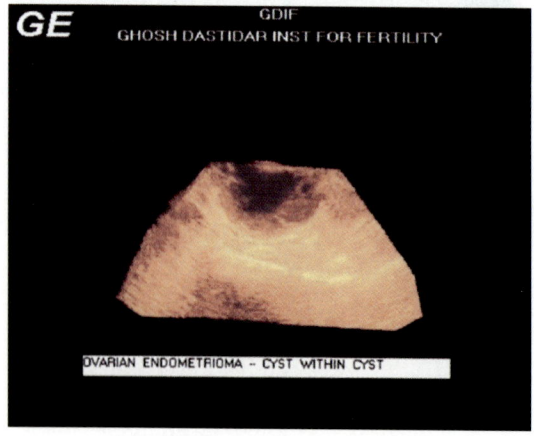

FIGURE 5.8: Cyst within cyst

found it difficult to believe. But after the arrival of 3D they take it more easily and on the other hand the woman carrying a normal baby finds it reassuring to see her baby.

3-Dimensional ultrasound has the advantage of taking very little time for acquisition of the picture. The patient spends very little time at the clinic. At a later period of time, the sonologist reconstructs the image using Cartesian storage technique and volume rendering and surface rendering to give a good picture from sections available in three planes exhibited at a time on the screen.

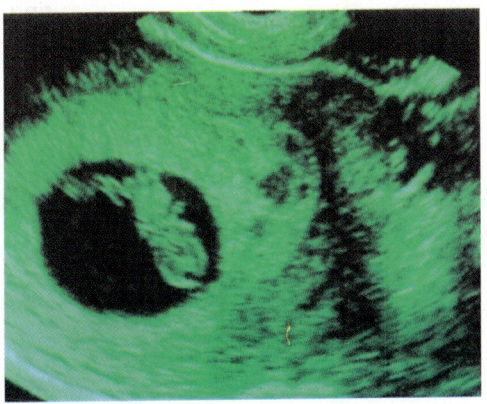

FIGURE 5.9: Umbilical cord and embryo
6 weeks—3D view

Chapter 6
Implantation

Ultrasound Confirms Implantation

The implanting trophoblast interacts with the decidua to alter the previously seen (layered) endometrial pattern which has also been studied by transvaginal sonography.

Embryo endometrial interaction within the milieu of the uterine cavity leading to implantation is an amazingly complex process. Among women expecting to get pregnant the expectation factor and anxiety is quite high in every such cycle. The anxiety increases manifold in patients being treated for infertility particularly those undergoing expensive Assisted Reproductive Technology (ART) programme. So early detection of healthy implantation can act as a factor to improve the psychological status of the recipient.

The existing concept of the foetus, as an allograft cherished by reproductive immunologist possibly needs reappraisal. The relationship between the allogenic conceptus and mother is possibly not governed by the laws of classical transplantation immunity; rather this interaction appears to be more akin to allorecognition system seen in invertebrates.

Human trophoblast in early stage of gestation has been seen to exhibit active cell locomotion, endocytosis and invasion of endometrial, cell monolayer in mixed cultures. This invasion requires action of proteolytic enzymes to degrade extra cellular matrix components of the endometrium. Matrix Metalloproteinases (MMPs) seem to be particularly important in this respect.

Whereas on the one hand pre-implantation factor (PIF) studied using lymphocyte/platelet binding assay in embryos could signify their capability to interact with the endometrium, on the other hand the necessity of the apical plasma membrane of the uterine epithelial cells to acquire adhesiveness is an essential prerequisite in embryo implantation. Studies in this area have indicated that modulation of a major element of the epithelial phenotype, i.e. apical basal cell polarity might be critical in this respect. Differential distribution of tight junctions like E-cadherin/plakoglobin complexes and E-cadherin/beta catenin complexes are correlated with the development of this apical adhesiveness of human uterine epithelial cells.

Integrin which are heterodymeric glycoprotein are a class of adhesion molecules that also participate in the cell-cell and cell-substratum interactions. They are expressed on the surface of all mammalian eggs and integrin alpha-6 beta-1 has been studied to serve as a sperm receptor; mediating sperm-egg binding. Beta-1 integrins are expressed on glandular epithelium in early proliferative phase and stromal cells in mid secretory phase of endometrium. The expression of beta-1 integrin increases at the time of implantation and disruption of the integrins expression has thus been reported to be associated with certain types of infertility in women. Varieties of cytokines have also been demonstrated at the placental-uterine interface.

Implantation followed by placenta formation is mainly based on two cell types, syncitiotrophoblast and cytotrophoblast which differentiate from the blastocyst wall derivative trophoblast cells, basically of epithelial origin. Cytotrophoblast cells lie in contact with the basal lamina and are the proliferating stem cells that guarantee persistence of both the cell types. Extra-villous trophoblasts exhibit strictly regulated invasiveness for maternal endometrial spiral arteries and dilate them in order to achieve sufficient foetal blood supply. These cells thus located in a remodeled uteroplacental artery wall are defined as intramural Cytotrophoblasts whose specific histochemical marker has been reported to be Cytokeratin 17. Studies done to detect variations in perfusion of human at microvascular level throughout the menstrual cycle using laser Doppler technique to assess red blood cell flux showed highest values at times associated with endometrial growth for preparation of implantation. At this stage of "invasion", c-Ttx 1 proto-oncogene has been suggested to play an important role in the angiogenesis occurring during the development of the villious tree.

Thus, the conceptus-mother crosstalk is accompanied by synchronization in interaction between the embryo and endometrium by local exchange of signals including a number of cytokines, growth factors, direct cell-cell and cell-matrix contact. However, though the research in early events of human implantation is still in its infancy significant studies at the cellular-biological-bio-chemical level have been done, but hardly any report on ultrasound studies of the phenomenon is on record.

When these biochemical-mediated histological sequences are in progress, the characteristic tissue perfusion at implantation site has been reported to be visible by high resolution ultrasound studies. Thus grey scale and Doppler study of "trophoblast migration" during implantation, i.e. as early as

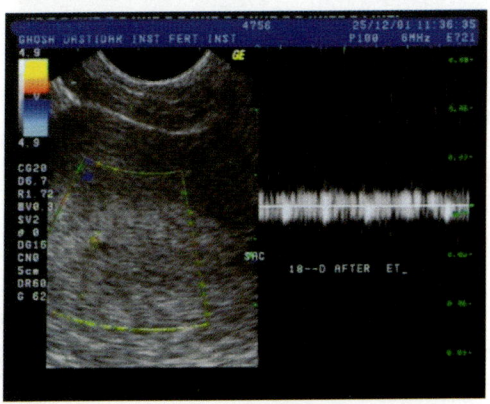

FIGURE 6.1: Early implantation flow parameter

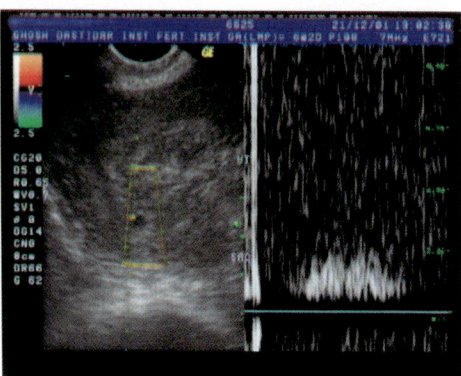

FIGURE 6.2: Gestational sac on 18D post-embryo transfer

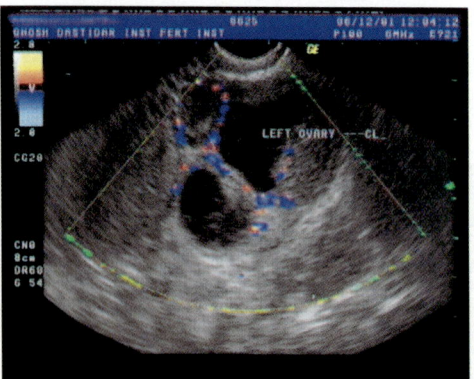

FIGURE 6.3: Corpus luteum—Ring of fire on CD

D-6 post transfer in IVF cycles reported by us seems to be a pioneer finding. The βhCG on day of scan for this study was around 16.4 mIU/ml (range 2.2 – 46.5 mIU/ml).

Chapter 7

Abnormal Stimulation and Other Ovulatory Disorders

Ovarian Hyperstimulation Syndrome (OHSS)

The only emergency side effect of controlled ovarian stimulation causing morbidity and mortality in the patient is hyperstimulation. The etiology is still unclear and has been attributed to growth of large number of follicles, very high velocity intraovarian blood flow with low resistance, accumulation of fluid in the peritoneal cavity, pleural effusion and even adult respiratory distress syndrome. Four varieties have been recognized. Whether the fluid is ovarian in origin is a doubt since extra peritonialization of ovary has not prevented fluid collection. At the moment vasoendothelial growth factor (VEGF) has been implicated to be a contributing factor. Patient having PCOD have been reported to be more prone to develop OHSS amongst them lean PCOS are worse than obese PCOS . In OHSS cycle the serum estradiol level is very high. Though specific treatment has not been evolved, withholding the administration of ovulation inducing human chorionic gonadotropin has been reported to prevent a full blown disease from occurring. The usual time when the patient comes with the complain is between 7 and 17 days following hCG injection. Pregnancy cycle in a patient with many follicles particularly cycle with multiple implantation have been seen to go into OHSS more frequently when undetected by prior ultrasound. Before giving hCG it becomes the sole

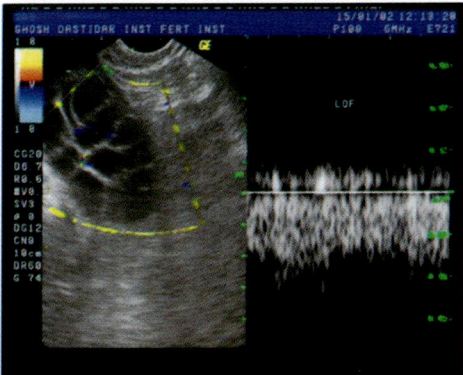

FIGURE 7.1: Moderate OHSS

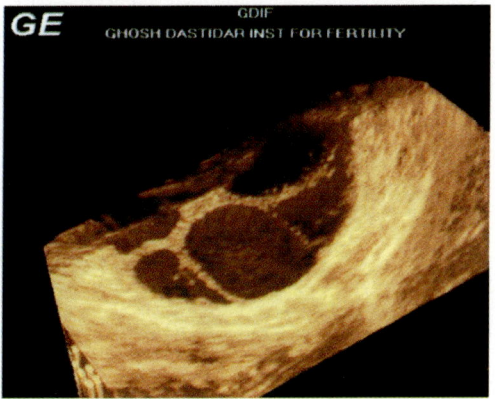

FIGURE 7.2: 3D view of OHSS

responsibility of the ultrasonologist to count the number of maturing follicles, measure their blood flow by colour Doppler, derive their follicular volume individually by 3D ultrasound and measure the POD fluid to prevent this life-threatening condition.

ENDOMETRIOSIS

Ultrasound Detects Endometriosis in very Early stage

Endometriosis is prevalent in approximately 15-25% of infertile patients. It might even occur earlier in reproductive life before infertility has been diagnosed, the patient usually coming with the complain of pain, dysmennorrhoea, dyspareunia or heaviness of lower abdomen. Strangely in most cases the symptoms are not associated with the severity of the disease. Many cases of unexplained infertility have been reported to be associated with

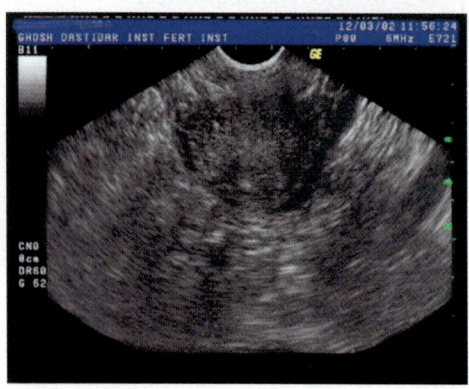

FIGURE 7.3: Early endometriotic deposits in ovary

early stage of pelvic endometriosis. Some patients are free of symptoms till quite late, when existing disease, with its associated pelvic adhesion gives rise to problem regarding treatment of disease and or restoration of fertility. At times this disease of yet unclear etiology affects only the deeper tissue of ovary. At this stage of preliminary disease the diagnosis is difficult since the complains are few. The staging is adversely affected immediately when such a lesion is of greater than 1 cm diameter and is classified stage III. In the early stage of deep seated pathology, laparoscopy is not effective diagnostically. The undiagnosed menace slowly bleeds itself to destruction and steadily damages the ovary and affects other area of pelvic tissue, the persistent cyclical haemorrhage also releases free iron, which is extensively fibrogenic giving rise

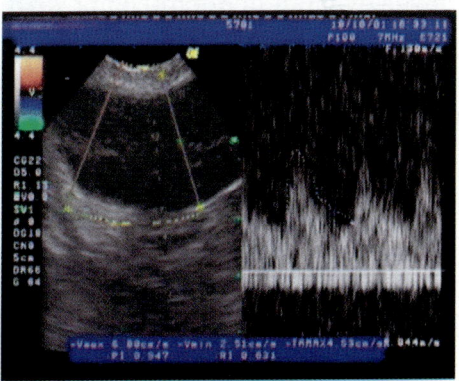

FIGURE 7.4: Chocolate cyst

to increasing grades of pelvic adhesion. Surgical treatment often gives rise to worser adhesions.

Medical treatment – hormonal therapy does not evoke excellent results for suppression of this ectopic functioning glandular tissue, possibly due to its altered nature of estrogen progesteron receptors. Many of these patients are advocated treatment with ART procedures which has been reported to give comparatively better result in terms of pregnancy outcome. Another method of surgical management – laser vaporization has also been reported to give good result. However all the above mentioned techniques are expensive and or invasive.

Pelvic ultrasonography is extremely efficient in diagnosing this disease in all its stages – (a) be it a small deep intraovarian sonolucent deposit or (b) very large ovarian endometrioma with typical internal echo, (c) small pelvic lesions or (d) adenomyotic ones are all easily diagnosed by pelvic sonography.

Polycystic Ovarian Disease

Polycystic ovarian disease is one of the most common endocrinopathies in women of reproductive age group but its etiology is still largely unknown. First described in 1721 by an Italian scientist Antonio Vallisneri, the syndrome was elaborated in 1935 by Stein and Leventhal in a group of hirsute, amennorrhoeic women on the basis of typical ovarian morphology; fibrotic thickening of tunica albuginea and outer cortex. Multiple cystic follicles with prominent theca was also described.

Though many of the patients come with complain of oligomennorrhoea, obesity, hirsutism, and infertility : many cases are asymptomatic to begin with. Here, ultrasound forms the backbone of diagnostic and therapeutic workup. On ultrasound– (1) large number of subcapsular small size cystic areas (2-8 mm), (2) enlarged ovarian diameter, (3) augmented ovarian volume measured by 3-D ultrasound, (4) hyperechoic ovarian stroma, (5) high velocity stromal blood flow with low resistance throughout cardiac cycle form the hallmark of diagnosis. Enhancement of ovarian volume takes place normally in female at 2 periods of life. (a) around 7 to 8 years of age, in response to circulating androgen, (b) at puberty due to rising level of gonadotropin and activity of growth hormone, insulin like growth factor-1 (IGF-1) and insulin. In patients suffering from PCOD the ovaries mostly enlarge irrespective of age. Recently Poretsky and Piper have postulated that elevated LH and hyperinsulinemia, acting synergistically, induce ovarian stromal and thecal hyperplasia, hyperandrogenism and follicular atresia.

Considering the complexity of the situation some authors believe PCOD to be just a sign of an underlying pathology. And others suggest familial inheritance with indication at autosomal dominant mode of inheritance. Though in a normal ovary the vascular flow indices fall through early follicular phase to reach lowest value in luteal phase, the flow in PCOD ovary, in contrast is of a bizarre pattern with low index value seen throughout the cycle. However, the vascular supply in the uterine artery of these patients shows increased resistance to blood flow – an effect which has been attributed directly to the vasoconstrictive action of elevated androstenedione level.

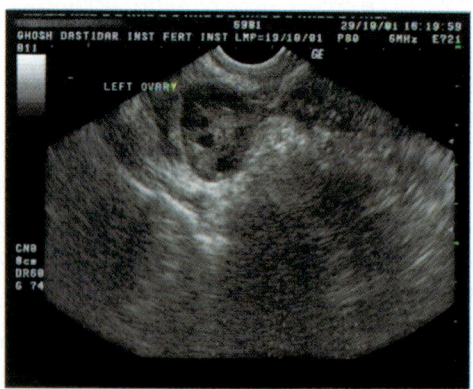

FIGURE 7.5: Polycystic ovary

Hyperinsulinaemia, insulin resistance, hyper-triglyceridemia are seen in PCO patients and they

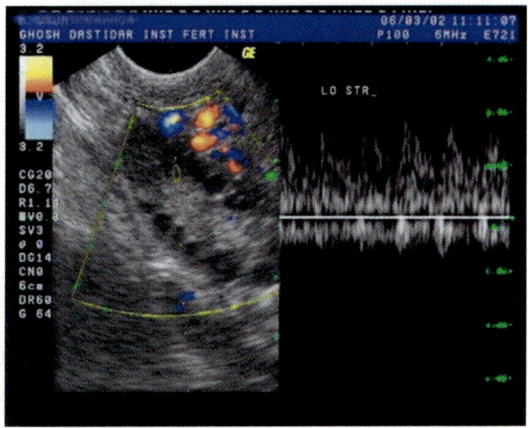

FIGURE 7.6: PCOD—Stromal flow

also show reduced isovolumetric relaxation of cardiac chambers in diastole with reduced ejection fraction. Some studies calculating risk factor for development of cardiovascular disease found an estimated 7-fold increase in PCOD patients. Enhanced coronary disease and atherosclerosis is also seen in them. They definitely form a high risk group for cardiovascular diseases. The question remains whether early recurrent miscarriages seen in PCOD patients is due to this different nature of uterine blood flow related to the above mentioned atherosclerotic change of uterine arteries. The low blood flow of the uterine artery seems to be of a similar mechanism to that of cardiovascular pathology.

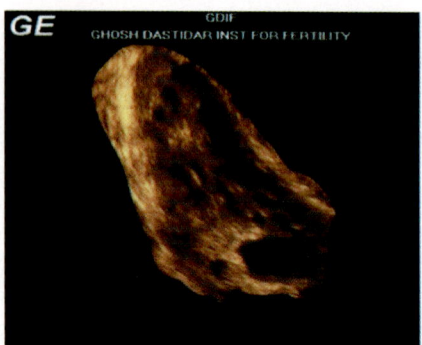

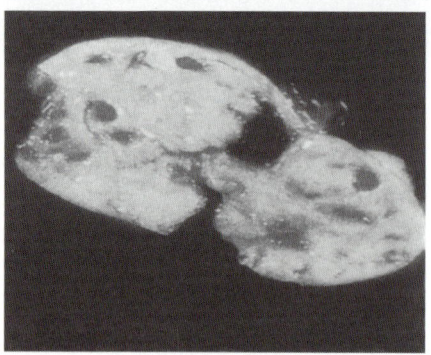

FIGURE 7.7: Compare cut surface of PCO ovary with 3D

Multifollicular Ovaries (MFO)

It is important to differentiate polycystic ovaries from multifollicular ovaries also presenting with ovarian cystic areas on ultrasound. MFO results from low levels of FSH stimulating partial folliculogenesis.

Biochemical parameters in such patients is normal. Using ultrasound the ovarian volume, stromal flow are seen to be normal and the cysts are fewer in number but larger in size (6-10 mm).

Chapter 8

Tubal Patency by Colour Doppler and 3D Ultrasound

To study endometrial cavity or fallopian tubes by 'Hystero-Sonosalpingography' saline infusion sonography is done. (Presently, developed centers are using 'Echovist' as contrast), however it is not available in market here.

STEPS OF SONOSALPINGOGRAPHY

After Basal Transvaginal Study

1. Patient is made to lie in lithotomy position with both legs on stirrups.
2. Antiseptic dressing is done (Drapings are done).
3. Vagina is cleaned with Povidone iodine solution.
4. Sim's speculum is introduced and the anterior lip of cervix is grasped with Allis' tissue forceps.
5. The cannula (HSG/Hydrotubation) is then introduced through the external os and lightly fixed.
6. In a sterile disposable syringe 50 cc of solution (normal saline) is drawn and fixed to the cannula.
7. During the examination, the patient must not be on full bladder (prior instructions given) and the sonologist now places the transvaginal transducer in the fornix, thus focusing the uterus and taking a look at the pelvic structures.

8. The assistant now injects 10 cc of fluid in a gradual fashion. Fluid is seen to distend the uterine cavity. (Linear echogenic filling).

9. Now the sonologist focuses the tubes one at a time on transverse scan. More fluid is injected. The fluid is seen to pass through each fallopian tube.

10. Remaining fluid is pushed by assistant and the slow trickle from the fimbrial ostium into the Pouch of Douglas is observed.

11. The patient is again observed by ultrasound 10 minutes later to note the volume of fluid collected in the Pouch of Douglas and the volume of fluid remaining in the uterine cavity. This is corroborated with the volume pushed by the assistant.

12. The whole procedure is done under colour Doppler and 3D guidance.

The patient is advised an antispasmodic in case of cramps in lower abdomen. The whole procedure is done under prior antibiotic cover.

If done around days 7-10 of cycle, best result is obtained and ovulatory studies can be combined. Endosalpingitis is diagnosed by 'Cogwheel Sign'.

Advantages of Sonosalpingography

a. Out-patient procedure.
b. No anaesthetic or radiation hazard.

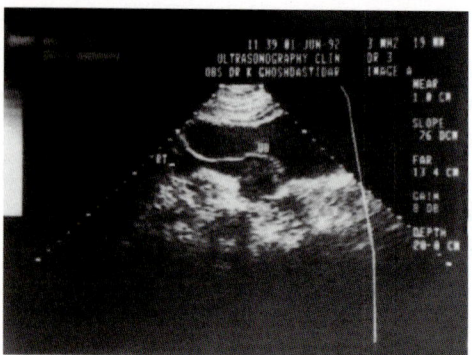

FIGURE 8.1: Dilated tube with terminal hydrosalpinx

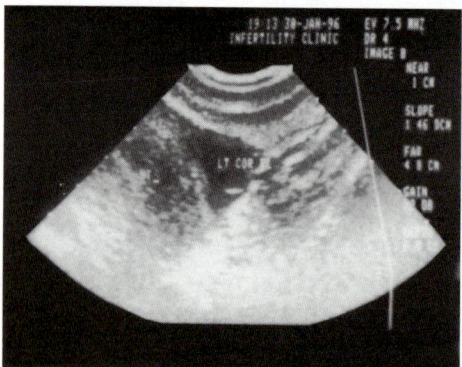

FIGURE 8.2: Cornual block

c. Easy, less expensive than laparoscopy.
d. Other pelvic pathology may be detected which is not so well discernable on HSG.
e. Follicular studies can be done at same time.

f. In cases of adhesions obliterating POD, chromotubation is not done during laparoscopy as the dye cannot be visualized. Most cases of adhesion can be seen by ultrasound.

g. No possibility of dye allergy (as in HSG).

h. Endometrium can be visualized.

i. Uterine cavity can be studied in detail.

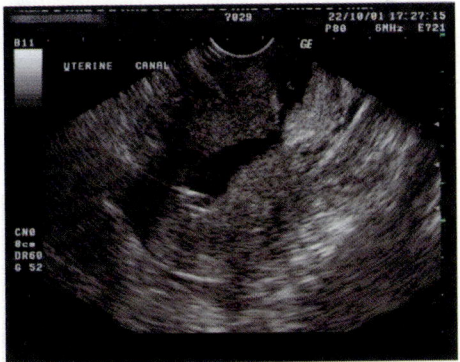

FIGURE 8.3: Uterine cavity during saline infusion

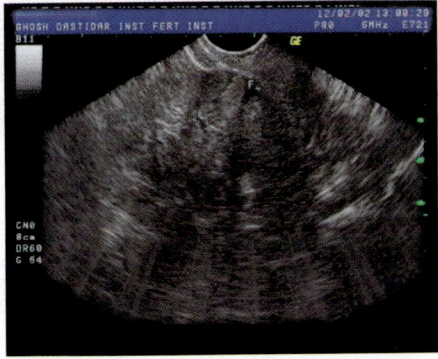

FIGURE 8.4: Fallopian tube and fimbria in 2D

Contraindication

1. Hydrosalpinx
2. Pelvic inflammatory disease.

Chapter 9

Obstetric Ultrasound

In normal pregnancies, ultrasound to be of benefit to the clinical situation two studies need generally be done:

a. One at around 14-16 weeks for evaluation of number of foetus, location of placenta, existing foetal anomaly, co-existing pelvic pathology.

b. At 30-32 weeks for monitoring growth pattern and confirmation of previous data.

Besides these, there are other clinical situations where an obstetric ultrasound is of benefit.

Focussing

Before starting the examination, it is essential to take the menstrual history and calculate the time since last menstrual period.

Optimally full bladder required for transvescical study. Focussing is done as described previously.

Empty bladder is required for first trimester transvaginal study.

Indications

First Trimester

1. Pain lower abdomen.
2. Bleeding per vaginum.
3. Abnormal uterine size as determined by bimanual palpation.
4. To re-confirm condition of already existing pelvic pathology.

5. Study the internal os, cervical canal in case of recurrent first trimester abortion.
6. For evaluation of foetal anatomical profile by transvaginal ultrasound in a patient who has delivered one or more congenitally anomalous foetus.
7. Following assisted reproductive procedure like IVF-ET, GIFT, etc. for evaluation of site and number of implantation to decide whether foetal reduction might be required or not.
8. Elderly women to rule out Trisomy 21 by Nuchal translucency.

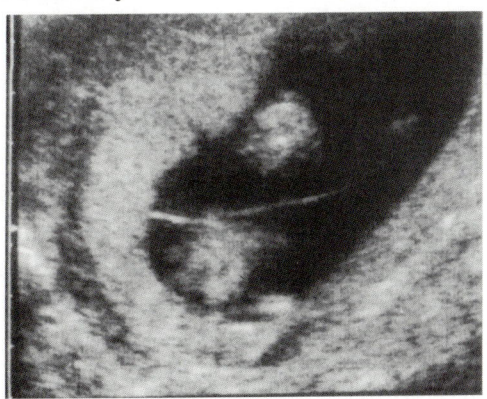

FIGURE 9.1: Twin monochorionic diamniotic

An operator in first trimester should look for:
a. Gestational sac
b. Identification of foetal pole.
c. Presence of cardiac activity and its rate.

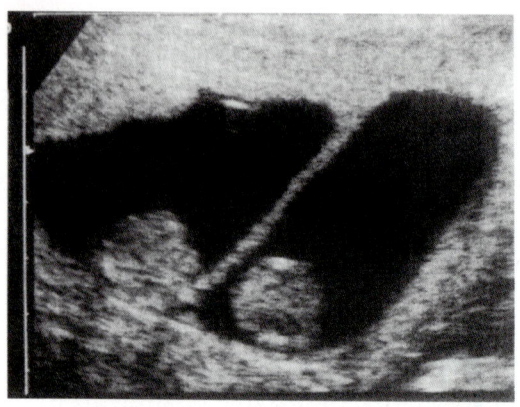

FIGURE 9.2: Twin peak sign—
Dichorionic diamniotic

d. Nature and frequency of foetal movement.
e. Location of chorion frondosum-decidua basalis complex.
f. Number of foetal echoes.
g. Presence and normalcy of yolk sac.
h. Crown rump length for age determination.

Second Trimester

a. Fetal viability
b. Amniotic fluid evaluation
c. Placental localization, character
d. Condition of cervix, os
e. Gestational age, anomaly

Third Trimester

a. Assessment of foetal growth,
b. Biophysical profile
c. Behavorial pattern,
d. Determination of foetal weight,
e. Reassessment of liquor volume and
f. Reconfirmation for absence of congenital anomaly done previously.

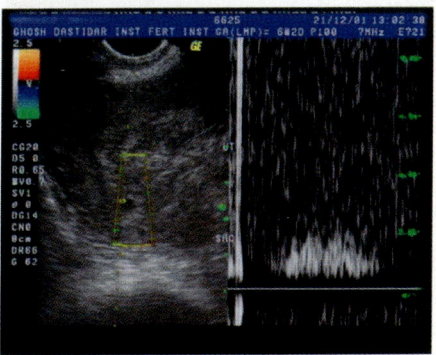

FIGURE 9.3: Gestational sac with choriodecidual blood flow—18D Post E.T.

ECTOPIC PREGNANCY

1.4% of all pregnancies are implanted outside the endometrial lining of uterine cavity of which 98% are within the fallopian tube.

Few causes that have been implicated for tubal implantation include congenital anomalies of fallopian tube like – diverticula, accessory ostia and

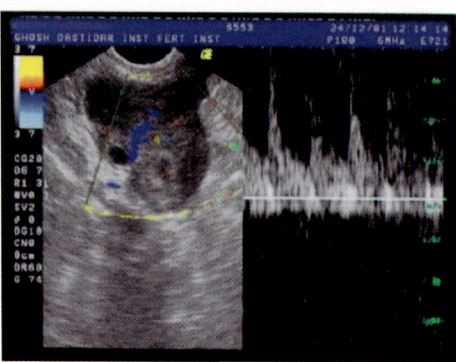

FIGURE 9.4: Tubal gestation with vascularity measurement of ectopic trophoblast

abnormal tubal length. Tubal pathologies in the form of endosalpingitis, endometriosis of endosalpinx or previous tubal infections are also significant causes. The above mentioned tubal pathologies are not visualized by 2D ultrasound unless the tube contains fluid. However, latest techniques like hysterosonosalpingography under 3D ultrasound guidance possibly forms the best method in the present time to diagnose such conditions. Other varieties of pelvic pathology that partially occlude the tubal lumen by external pressure and cause impaired tubal motility may result in tubal implantation. Rarer sites of ectopic implantation include the ovary, cervix or anywhere in the abdominal cavity.

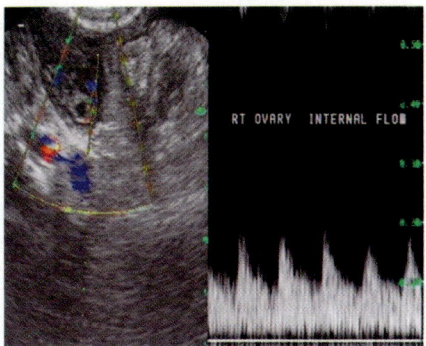

FIGURE 9.5: Ovarian pregnancy

Increased incidence of ectopic gestation has been reported in IUCD users and those on low dose progesterone which is thought to alter endocrine milieu of tubal lumen. Ectopic pregnancy accounts for 15% of maternal mortality, morbidity. In undetected cases the maternal mortality increases 10-fold when compared to a normal vaginal delivery. Its incidence among infertile patients has also been quite high which could be due to tubal factor common to both situations. Advent of infertility management has increased heterotopic implantation from 1 in 30,000 to nearly 1 in 7,000. **The classical clinical triad of pain, vaginal bleeding and adnexal mass is not present in all the patients.** Delayed diagnosis complicates maternal condition. Ultrasound can diagnose ectopic pregnancy in very early stage by (1) locating the ectopic sac with or

without cardiac activity, (2) locating empty endometrial cavity with thickened hyperechoic endometrium containing some fluid – "Pseudo decidual
reaction" in a case of positive biochemical
pregnancy —even when the ectopic sac is not very
well visualized, (3) locating an intrauterine sac
which does not show any embryo (an embryonic
pregnancy), disturbed gestational status with
irregular sac outline and open cervical canal
(inevitable abortion). In the last case the complain
of pain, bleeding is attributed to the intrauterine
disturbed pregnancy and not to ectopic gestation
unless it is due to rare case of heterotopic
pregnancy, (4) fluid collection in the fallopian tube
and POD – tubal abortion.

SONOEMBRYOLOGY CALENDAR

A fruitful obstetric study can never be done if the
obstetric time-table or happenings are not appreciated by the operator. In brief, ovulation, in a natural
cycle takes place 14 days prior to the next cycle.
Fertilisation takes place within approximately 24
hours of **ovulation** to form the **zygote** which gets
completely implanted, by D-23 of an approximately
4 weeks cycle. From here till the 10th week it is
known as the **embryo.** The endometrium that had
been *proliferating* under the endocrine influence
of the cycle, becomes *secretory* and embedding

blastocyst burrows through this endometrium which then gets sealed off. The fluid filled cavity or blastocyst cavity of the embryo is visualized as the anechoic sac at 4th week. As the extraembryonic coelom develops the primary yolk sac is pinched off and extruded resulting in the formation of secondary yolk sac which is actually visible on ultrasound around 5th week with transvaginal scanning (TVUS). At times the yolk sac is only seen and foetal pole is not yet visualized. The yolk sac has a diameter of 3 to 6 mm throughout its presence. It is essential to study the yolk sac, measure its diameter and wall thickness. It has been reported that enhanced thickening of the wall has been associated with a congenitally anomalous foetus at later gestational age. Sometimes too thin a wall has been reported to be associated with spontaneous abortion. In the presence of a healthy yolk sac, even when foetal pole is not demonstrable, further studies have revealed a healthy growing foetus.

Towards the end of the 5th weeks of gestational age the formation of the neural plate and neural tube takes place. From the cephalic end of the tube the brain vesicle formation starts towards this time. Failure of completion of the neural tube causes deformities with resultant increament of maternal serum alpha fetoprotein.

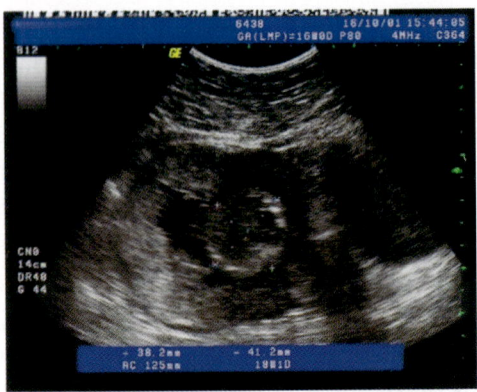

FIGURE 9.6: Measuring foetal parameters—
AC (Abdominal circumference)

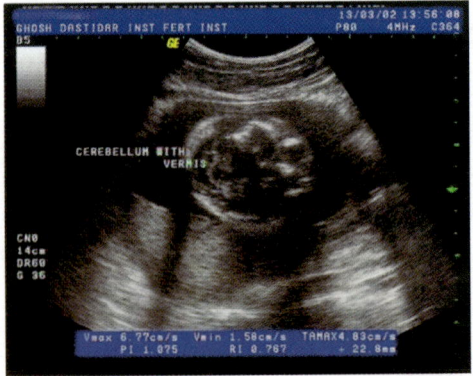

FIGURE 9.7: Intercerebellar distance

Alpha Fetoprotein (AFP)

First detected in human foetal serum in 1956, it
has a molecular weight of 68,000 daltons and is
therefore, small enough to cross the placenta. It

is normally virtually undetectable in the adult except in the presence of certain types of tumour but is detectable in foetal serum and is at peak approximately at 13-14 weeks of gestation (3 mg/ml), thereafter falling rapidly at birth (cord serum). Aminotic fluid concentration follows a similar pattern but is 100-200 times less per unit volume, where its chief source is foetal urine in midtrimester. But in contrast the maternal serum AFP rises in concentration throughout pregnancy reaching a peak at 30 weeks. At 16 weeks the concentration is about 30 mg /ml.

SONOEMBRYOLOGY

At the beginning of the 6th weeks the prosencephalon cleaves to form the telencephalon and diencephalons. Telecephalon gives rise to brain hemispheres and the lateral ventricle and falx cerebri. Improper cleavage here will give rise to holoprosencephaly.

At this time there is also the formation of two cardiac tubes which are functional in a smooth contractile fashion visible by ultrasound from the end of 5th week. In fact, it is the first organ to reach a functioning state.

The alimentary system starts formation around the 6th week and due to rapid growth of liver dorsally and stomach ventrally the midgut herniates into the umbilical cord from the 8th week and returns into the abdomen around 11th week. Anomaly of this phenomenon and abdominal wall formation results in :

1. Umbilical hernia
2. Omphalocoele
3. Gastroschisis, all of which are visible clearly by ultrasound.

The limb buds form from 5th week and can be studied by TVUS from 7th to 8th week and even at 10th week the soles of feet face medially and hands are laid ventrally.

The ureteric bud and metanephros give rise to the kidneys at 6th weeks. Then the kidneys ascend from the pelvis towards their anatomical site, the process starting in the 8th week and is complete by the 11th week. The kidneys start producing urine around the 11-12th weeks of gestation, when it can be recorded by ultrasound.

At 9 weeks a thin plate of cranial bone begins to be seen and ossification of the skeletal system starts. At this stage the cranium is seen to be filled with echogenic choroid plexuses which gradually diminishes in size. By the 10th week the foetus attains the human look. It is during the period of time discussed above that disturbances of embryo-genesis results in congenital malformations except those of the external genitalia which remain in a sexless state here.

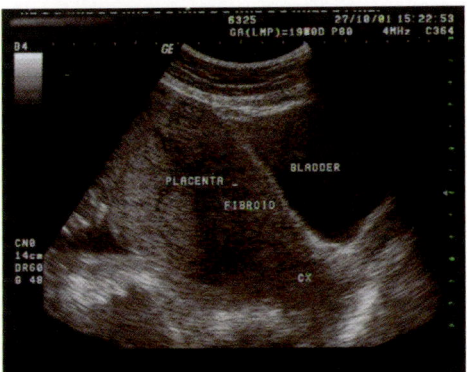

FIGURE 9.8: Placenta praevia

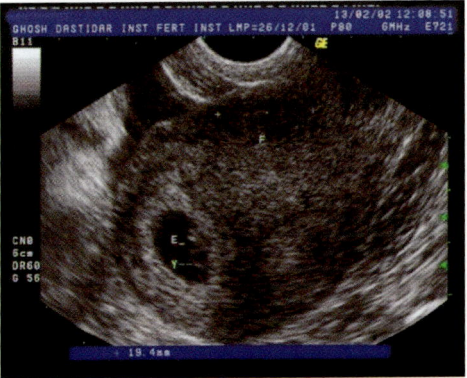

FIGURE 9.9: Pregnancy with fibroid (F)

Over 200 different abnormalities have till now been diagnosed *in utero* by ultrasound. Campbell & Smith have pioneered this diagnostic ability and suggest that the optimum time for obstetrics screening is 14 to 16 weeks.

Chapter 10

Foetal Biometry

For determination of foetal age first trimester scan is most dependable when it measures the crown rump length (CRL) valid upto 12 weeks. At 8 weeks of gestation the diameter of yolk sac equals to the diameter of head. Some studies also use the diameter of gestational sac for pregnancy dating. However, since usually ultrasound is done later than the first trimester, parameters used for foetal age and growth monitoring include :

1. Biparietal diameter (BPD),
2. Femur length (FL),
3. Intercerebellar diameter,
4. Length of other long bones like humerus, radius, tibia,
5. Length of the sole of foot,
6. Inter orbital distance

Growth and Weight is usually monitored by:

a. Head circumference (HC)
b. Abdominal circumference (AC)
c. Ratio of HC/AC
d. Femur length

The advent of 3-Dimensional ultrasound offers a number of potentially important advantages for biometry. The procedure is more accurate and reliable due to improved definition of landmarks and by ability to measure true volume.

Normal Anatomy

A systematic approach to sonographic examination of the fetal structures is necessary to reveal the numerous possible abnormalities in this complex system along with growth/age determination.

Head

The foetal head is most often in an occiput-transverse position (i.e. the side of the head lies parallel to the mother's abdominal wall).

The Lateral Ventricles

The lateral ventricles are identified as paired echo-spared areas within the brain substance. The distal ventricle (i.e. the one farthest from the ultrasound transducer) is chosen for study, as reverberation artifacts often obscure the anatomy of the proximal hemisphere. A prominent echogenic area is often seen within the lateral ventricle, which represents the choroid plexus.

The Biparietal Diameter

Perhaps the most intensely studied transverse section of the fetus is at the level of the biparietal diameter (BPD). Several intracranial landmarks are located at a plane 15° above the canthomeatal line and parallel to the base of the skull. The two landmarks most consistently found are the roughly triangular, paired, non-echogenic thalami and two short anterior lines parallel to the midline, known as the cavum septi pellucidi. Other structures commonly observed in the same plane and near the midline are from posterior to anterior : the great cerebral vein and its ambient cistern sitting above the cerebellum, the midbrain, the third ventricle between the thalami, and the frontal horns of the lateral ventricles. Laterally placed, in the same plane, are the spiral hippocampal gyri posteriorly and the bright paired echoes of the insulae with pulsating middle cerebral arteries, commonly studied for velocimetry since it is comparatively easy to focus.

In this plane, the BPD can be reproducibly measured as the distance from the proximal outer table to the distal inner table of the skull. In addition, the head perimeter can be determined by direct measurement or calculated by summing the BPD and occipito-frontal diameter (OFD) measured from the midpoint of frontal and occipital echo complexes and multiplying by 1.62. The ratio of BPD to OFD defines the cephalic index (normal values 75-85). A high value determines brachycephaly and a low value dolicocephaly.

The Cerebellum

The cerebellum may be visualized in a plane parallel to the BPD plane with posterior angulation.

Once located, the cerebellar structures are best studied by rotating the ultrasound transducer 15^0 farther from the cantho-meatal line. In this plane, the cerebellum (with its brightly echogenic, centrally-placed vermis, and two relatively non-echogenic hemispheres) may be evaluated and measured.

The Base of the Skull

The base of the skull level may be identified by an echogenic 'X' formed by the lesser wings of the sphenoid bone and the petrous pyramid. These bone ridges mark the anterior, middle and posterior fossae.

The Face

Unlike the cranium and its contents, which may be studied using an orderly progression of well-defined sonographic planes, characterization of the face requires both ingenuity and good luck on the part of the sonographer. 3-D ultrasound is invaluable to study the face.

The Ears

The pinna of the ear and the development of its cartilages have been observed sonographically.

The Lower Face

The nose and the upper lip can be visualized using an oblique transverse scan. This plane may be used in the search for cleft lip and cleft palate.

Foetal Weight

Abdominal circumference calculated from two orthogonal abdominal diameters at level of intrahepatic portion of umbilical vein and stomach along with BPD computes foetal weight. Many formulas have been formulated by different workers for estimation of foetal weight. However the exact weight is not obtained by any. The accuracy of weight prediction comes with a relative error which is the difference between estimated and actual weights, expressed as fraction of actual weight.

From a large study of 12,980 obstetric cases the following values of foetal parameters were calculated in the author's ultrasound laboratory.

Foetal Growth Retardation

Foetal intrauterine growth retardation (IUGR) or foetal growth retardation and oligo-hydramnios in second half of pregnancy, may complicate 1% of all pregnancies and indicate poor prognosis for the

Table 10.1: Median (M) and 5th, 95th estimated centiles for fetal femur length (FL) in mm per gestational age

Weeks	FL VALUES		
	5th	M	95th
20	28	34	40
21	30	37	43
22	32	40	46
23	35	43	49
24	37	45	52
25	39	47	54
26	42	49	57
27	44	52	59
28	45	54	61
29	49	56	63
30	51	58	65
31	54	61	67
32	56	63	69
33	58	65	70
34	60	67	72
35	62	69	74
36	63	71	76
37	64	73	78
38	65	74	79
39	66	75	80

Table 10.2: Median (M) and 5th, 95th estimated centiles for fetal head circumference (HC) in mm per gestational age.

Weeks	HC VALUES		
	5th	M	95th
20	143	174	190
21	154	183	212
22	162	196	217
23	176	206	235
24	184	217	243
25	199	231	265
26	214	241	268
27	216	248	269
28	217	259	295
29	229	272	306
30	249	278	306
31	256	284	312
32	260	291	315
33	263	300	320
34	271	304	322
35	286	313	328
36	290	314	332
37	294	317	339
38	299	319	343
39	300	322	347

Table 10.3: Median (M) and 5th, 95th estimated centiles for fetal biparietal diameter (BPD) in mm per gestational age.

Weeks	BPD VALUES		
	5th	M	95th
20	38	47	54
21	42	50	59
22	44	53	63
23	47	56	66
24	50	59	68
25	53	62	72
26	55	65	74
27	58	67	76
28	61	71	81
29	64	74	83
30	67	76	83
31	69	78	85
32	70	79	87
33	74	83	90
34	76	84	91
35	79	85	91
36	79	86	91
37	80	87	93
38	81	87	93
39	81	89	94

Table 10.4: Median (M) and 5th, 95th estimated centiles for fetal occipito-frontal diameter (OFD) in mm per gestational age.

Weeks	OFD VALUES		
	5th	M	95th
20	53	61	69
21	55	65	76
22	58	69	80
23	67	73	86
24	69	78	89
25	70	82	93
26	72	83	96
27	78	87	99
28	80	96	110
29	82	99	111
30	88	100	113
31	90	102	115
32	92	104	116
33	94	106	116
34	95	108	117
35	97	109	118
36	99	110	119
37	100	113	122
38	103	113	124
39	103	114	127

Table 10.5: Median (M) and 5th, 95th estimated centiles for fetal abdominal circumference (AC) in mm per gestational age.

Weeks	AC VALUES		
	5th	M	95th
20	108	151	165
21	122	162	180
22	135	170	190
23	144	180	205
24	155	189	221
25	168	200	228
26	182	211	238
27	191	219	255
28	195	231	273
29	207	243	279
30	216	251	287
31	224	262	299
32	234	268	306
33	241	277	313
34	246	286	323
35	252	291	330
36	257	293	331
37	266	300	335
38	276	311	345
39	284	320	356

Table 10.6: Median (M) and 5th, 95th estimated centiles for the ratio of head and abdominal circumferences (HC/AC) x 100, per gestational age.

Weeks	*HC/AC VALUES (× 100)*		
	5th	*M*	*95th*
20	109	119	135
21	103	117	133
22	101	117	132
23	100	117	132
24	99	115	132
25	98	115	131
26	97	115	130
27	96	112	130
28	95	111	128
29	95	111	126
30	95	110	126
31	94	109	124
32	94	108	124
33	94	108	121
35	94	106	119
36	94	106	117
37	93	104	114
38	92	102	114
39	92	102	113

foetus. Probably low birth weight is, not only the single most important determinant of neonatal mortality but is also a significant contributing factor to post-neonatal infant mortality and childhood morbidity. When other causes of foetal compromise such as foetal congenital anomaly is an associated feature, the rate of foetal mortality is quite high. Even when normal foetuses are exposed to the adversity of growth retardation and oligohydramnios a mortality of 6 out of 7 was recorded in one study.

Though a large percentage of foetal growth retardation is associated with maternal PIH, no cause is apparent in a good percentage of cases. It has been suggested that some of these growth retarded fetuses with no apparent cause of IUGR are chronically hypoxic. In normal intrauterine gestations, migration of trophoblast into spiral arteries cause characteristic progressive increment in diastolic flow through feto-placental circulation with resultant decrease in peak systolic to diastolic flow ratio, Pulsatility Index (PI). In fetal growth retardation elevation of placental vascular resistance has been suggested since vascular studies have shown to have decreased umbilical artery diastolic flow and increased PI values. Thus resulting in placental insufficiency.

For assessment of pre-eclampsia and IUGR; evaluation of vascular flow parameters of uterine artery by Doppler ultrasound has shown promising results. This branch of internal iliac artery arising close to the bifurcation of common iliac shows progressive decrease of flow impedance in pregnancy, possibly due to trophoblast migration of spiral arteries during implantation and thereof until approximately 24 weeks. RI and PI are both measured during gestational studies. Early diastolic notching, absent diastolic flow or reversal of end diastolic flow detected in mid-second trimester has been reported to be associated with development of pre-eclampsia, foetal growth retardation, placental abruption and foetal death in the third trimester. High PI values between 23-27 weeks of gestation are ten times more likely to deliver preterm in comparison with those women showing normal PI value in uterine artery.

This placental insufficiency resultant from abnormal trophoblastic invasion of the maternal spiral arteries exposes the foetus to an environment of chronic hypoxia. Foetal blood velocity studies have been suggested to be more sensitive than cardiotocography in detecting foetal hypoxia. Such hypoxic fetuses have been treated *in utero* with maternal inhalation of humidified oxygen (55-60%) through face-mask. Oxygen inhalation has been reported to result in sustained increase in blood velocity and improved foetal outcome.

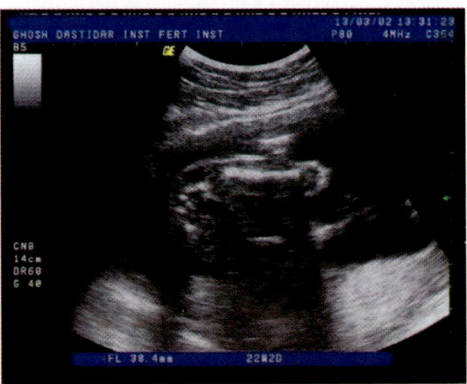

FIGURE 10.1: Measurement of foetal femur for determination of age

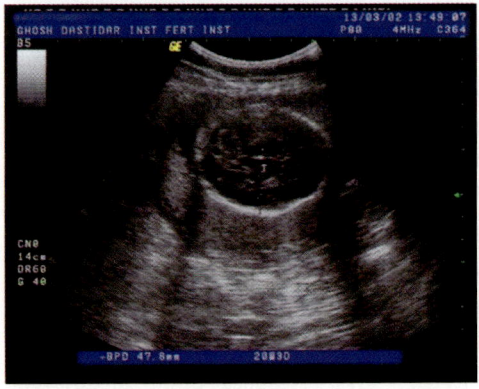

FIGURE 10.2: Measurement of biparietal diameter (BPD)

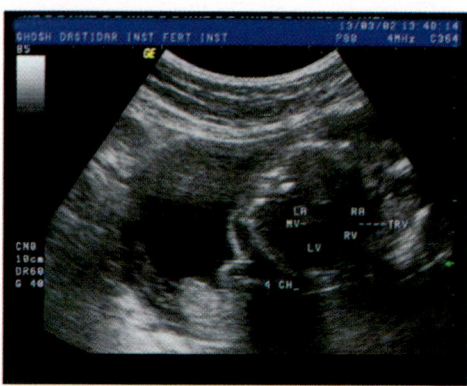

FIGURE 10.3: Detailed study of heart

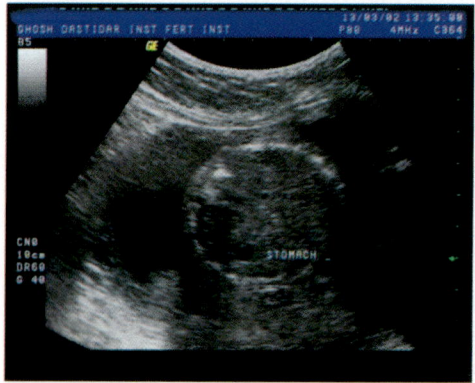

FIGURE 10.4: Detailed study of stomach

In a significant number of cases of foetal growth retardation, no primary maternal, or foetal cause can be implicated. The vascular flow indices in such cases show poor diastolic flow and increased resistive indices. It has been shown that maternal inhalation of moist oxygen improves these flow parameters, measured by vascular Doppler studies. Resultant foetal growth improvement reduces; foetal/neonatal morbidity/mortality significantly. However, all cases treated thus, do not respond positively hence very close monitoring of flow patterns and foetal weight gain need to be done by serial ultrasound study.

Chapter 11

Congenital Anomalies

Congenital anomaly is defined as an anatomical abnormality present at birth due to

a. embryological malformation
b. deformation due to abnormal intrauterine mechanical constraint, e.g. amniotic band sequence
c. disruption after normal formation
d. dysplasia or disorganization of specific tissue type.

Congenital anomaly—may be

- Major
- Minor variety.

Major   Those that produce long-term disability and or death.

Minor   Compatible with life.
   All anomalies are not detectable at birth.

Incidence of Individual Anomalies

Since majority of severe anomalies are incompatible with growth/life embryonic death occurs early and over 50% first trimester abortus show chromosomal anomalies. Only 0.5-0.7% of live births shows major chromosomal anomaly which in order of incidence are :

Cardiovascular	– 34.4%
Musculoskeletal	– 25.2%
Central nervous system	– 16.8%

Oro-facial	– 12.8%
Gastrointestinal	– 3.6%
Abdominal wall defect	– 2.8%
Pulmonary	– 2.5%
Genitourinary	– 1.8%

Five Major Causes of Malformation are Recognised

1. Chromosome abnormality—6%
2. Single gene disorder—8%
3. Teratogenic (environmental)—7% (drug or chemical, infectious agent, radiation, metabolic, e.g. glucose metabolism)
4. Combined or multifactorial—25%
5. Unknown—54%

In Terms of Vulnerable Phase

Day 15- 65 post-conception is important, however when the cause in maternal hyperglycaemia periconceptional period is important.

Drug or Chemical Agent as Potential Cause of Malformation

- Alcohol
- Acetazolamide
- Amitriptyline
- Amobarbital
- Azathioprine
- Caffeine
- Captopril
- Carbamazepine

- Chlordiazepoxide
- Chloroquine
- Chlorpropamide
- Clomiphene
- Cocaine
- Codeine
- Cortison
- Coumadine
- Cyclophosphamide
- Daunorubicin
- Dextroamphetamine
- Diazepam
- Diuretics
- Disulfiram
- Estrogen
- Ethosuccimide
- Fluorouracil
- Haloperidol
- Imipramine
- Indomethacin
- Isoniazid
- Methotrexate
- Metronidazole
- Nortriptyline
- OC pills
- Phenobarbitol
- Phenothiazines
- Phenylephrine
- Phenytoin
- Quinine
- Retinoic acid
- Sulfonamide
- Tetracycline
- Thalidomide
- Thioguanine
- Tobacco
- Tolbutamide
- Trimethadione
- Valproic acid

MAJOR ANOMALIES OF CENTRAL NERVOUS SYSTEM

1 Anencephaly (Skeletal)
2. Hydrocephalus
3. Meningocele
4. Hydranencephaly.

Brain development : 6-18 menstrual weeks.

Three primary segments of proximal neural tube gives rise to 5 secondary segments. They are as follows (Table 11.1):

Table 11.1

Forebrain (Prosencephalon)	Telencephalon Diencephalon
Midbrain (Mesencephalon)	Mesencephalon Metencephalon
Hindbrain (Rhombencephalon)	Myelecephalon

The wall and the cavity of the segments give rise to the following:

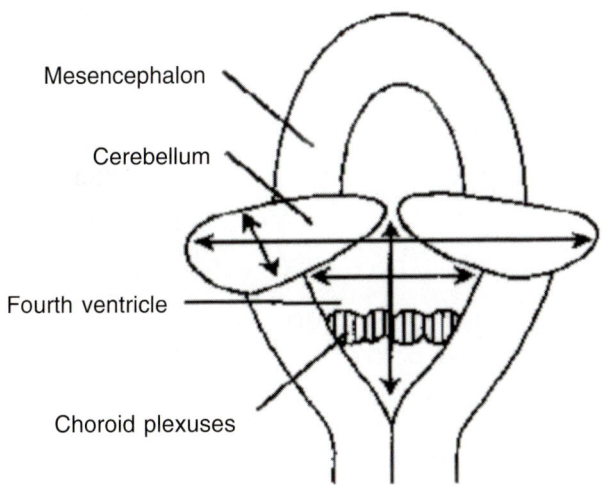

Mesencephalon

Cerebellum

Fourth ventricle

Choroid plexuses

FIGURE 11.1: Development of posterior mesencephalon and rhombencephalon

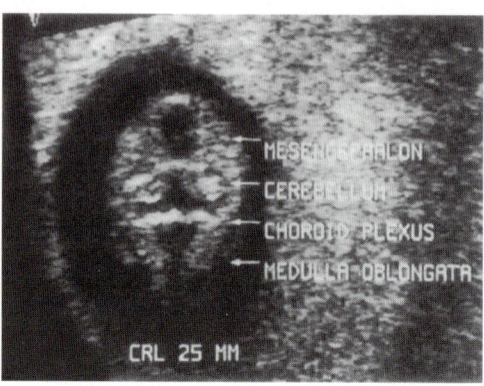

FIGURE 11.2: Coronal section through hindbrain—Ultrasound view

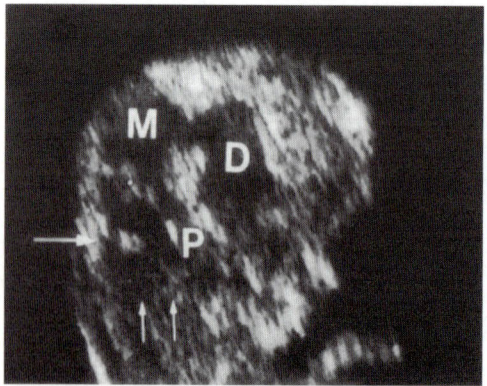

FIGURE 11.3: Ultrasound view—Sagittal section of brain at 12 weeks. D—Diencephalon, M—Mesencephalon, P—Medulla, pons

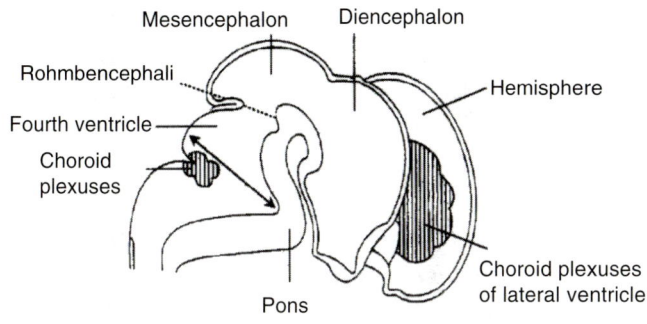

FIGURE 11.4: Sagittal section through developing brain

Derivatives

Walls		Cavities
Cerebral hemisphere (Failure to develop give rise to holoprosencephaly)	Telencephalon	Lateral ventricle
Thalami	Diencephalon	Third ventricle
Midbrain	Mesencephalon	Aqueduct
Pons, cerebellum	Metencephalon	Upper and lower part of 4th ventricle
(Dandy-Walker malformation results from agenesis of cerebellum).		
Medulla	Myelencephalon	Spinal canal

MUSCULOSKELETAL

Skeletal dysplasias are a rare and heterogeneous group of anomalies which are usually genetically determined.

International nomenclature for skeletal dysplasia subdivides the anomalies into 5 groups.

1. Osteochondrodysplasia—Abnormality of cartilage or bone growth/development.
2. Dysostoses—Malformations of individual bones singly or in combination.
3. Idiopathic osteolyses — Disorders associated with multifocal reabsorption of bone.
4. Skeletal disorders associated with chromosomal aberrations.
5. Primary metabolic disorders.

Limb/Long Bone Disorder

1. Shortening :
   Proximal segment —Rhizomelic
   Intermediate segment—Mesomelic
   Distal segment—Acromelic
   All segments—Micromelic
2. Excessive long bone curvature — Campomelia
3. Altered echotexture for mineralization disturbance hypophosphatasia.
4. Alteration in number, size, shape, position of fingers, toes.

GENITOURINARY

Edith L Potter worked extensively on foetal renal pathology and the diseases are named after her.

1. Potter type I—Autosomal recessive polycystic kidney.
2. Potter type II —Multicystic/dysplastic kidney disease.
3. Potter type III—Autosomal dominant polycystic kidney.
4. Potter type IV—Cystic kidneys due to urethral obstruction.

CARDIOVASCULAR

Out of all foetuses born with congenital anomalies the largest number have defects in the cardiovascular system.

Seventy to eighty percent of congenital anomalies can be excluded from 4-chambered view of heart.

GASTROINTESTINAL

Normally physiological gut herniation is not visible at 12 weeks of gestation by which time rotation of gut makes it re-enter abdomen.

Foetal stomach is visible at 11th week.

By second trimester bowel loops should be visible.

Obstruction commonly due to atresia is at level of:
a. Esophagus
b. Pylorus
c. Duodenum

d. Lower intestine
e. Colonic.

Frequent Anomalies of GI System

- Omphalocele
- Gastroschises
- Congenital diaphragmatic hernia
- Cloacal and bladder extrophy.

EARLY SCREENING FOR FOETAL ANOMALY

Well as of today the sonologist's view is something like the third umpire in a game of cricket – Omnipresent. But behold ! we shall come to it later.

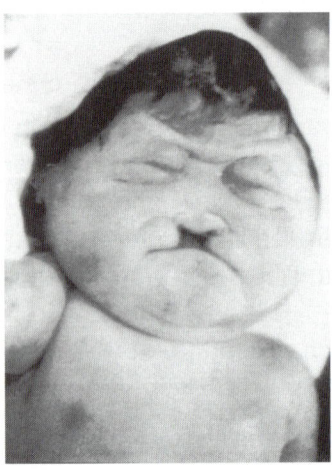

FIGURE 11.5: Bilateral cleft lip with skeletal dysplasia

Let us visualise the expectant family first who have been eagerly waiting and might have also decided a name for the baby, may be some distant relatives have arrived for the birth. And the baby is born who looks like this (Fig. 11.5) or the sono-logist has reported that the foetus is anomalous during a scan late in pregnancy. The unwilling couple with some disbelief agrees to undergo MTP and a baby is born with abdominal contents jutting out; deformed face and extremities and it gives a shock to the parents. In a study Prof Schuth of Frieberg Germany comments that the parents become apprehensive, self reproachful and scared of having another baby. Prof David Nyberg, one of the authorities on congenital anomalies says the Psychosocial life of the parents change completely after an anomalous birth.

Anomalies are detected in 2-5% of newborns and account for 20-30% perinatal demise. In actuality the incidence in nature is much higher but since the more lethal anomalies are incompatible even at early gestation, a large percentage end in foetal demise. Thus about **50%** of 1st trimester abortus are chromosomally abnormal.

In the United States of America alone **1 Lakh 50 Thousand** congenitally malformed neonates are born yearly. However, there being no such registry in our country we do not have the exact number of such cases **but does that matter?**

Every anomalous child born in the expectant family comes as a shock and changes the psychosocial life of the parents.

Anomalous conditions ammenable to treatment in live neonates are highly expensive, so much so that the pioneer in ultrasound **Prof Stuart Campbell** feels that "such early neonatal care far exceeds a man's life time earning".

The earlier such conditions are detected *in utero* the better it is for the parents and doctors. Previously done biochemical studies were invasive and have been steadily overtaken by ultrasound diagnosis over the last few years. Maternal serum alfa feto-protein, and amniotic fluid AFP were raised in some anomalies, particularly of the neural tube. But these also give false-positives in multiple gestation, in inaccurate pregnancy dating, missed abortion and technical failure. Maternal serum alfa fetoprotein (MSAFP) first detected in 1972 by Prof Brock in neural tube defect (NTD) is raised or lowered in different foetal anomalies. However, since the test for MSAFP or amniocentesis is

1. Invasive
2. Can only be done quite late in pregnancy, around **16-18 weeks** when foetal cells can be available and 2 more weeks are required for cell culture, it gets quite late till the result is obtained for any decision like MTP to be taken in case the foetus is diagnosed to be anomalous.

3. False-positive in multiple gestation, missed abortion, etc and

4. Abortion rate due to procedure like amniocentesis is quite high — **.2 - .5%,** it is no longer a method of choice anymore.

Ultrasound can detect major anomalies much earlier. The superiority of present day ultrasound technology and experience has allowed vision of unsurpassed clarity into the pregnant uterus very early in gestation. Advent of transvaginal sonography (TVS- 7.5 MHz), Colour Doppler, 3D Ultrasound has improved noninvasive detection of physiological function and pathologies in the body which includes those in pelvis and foetus.

Embryological developments taking place from 5th week follows through 12th week for all organs and upto 18th weeks of gestation for brain. Unless the knowledge about normal structural growth or formation (embryology) is clear, it is difficult to appreciate malformation in different organs. Knowledge of some embryology has thus become imperative for sonologist involved in foetal study. **In terms of vulnerable phase for anomaly development :** Day 15-65 post-conception is important, however when the cause in maternal hyperglycaemia periconceptional period is important. Most organs formed by 8th week are visible by the **Transvaginal** (7.5 MHz) study. Newer additions like Colour Doppler, Pulsed Doppler, 3D and 4D is constantly improving diagnostic accuracy. However it is important to remember that repeat study after 5-6 days is essential before commenting on anomaly.

G.D.Inst. Fert. Res.

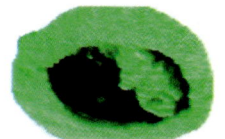

8W Embryo - 3D View

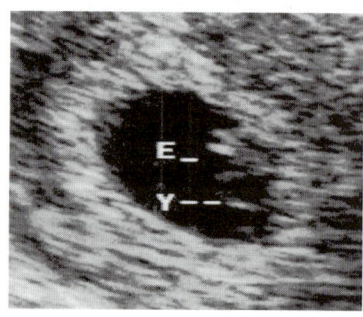

FIGURE 11.6: Eight weeks embryo and yolk sac

Ultrasound Markers

1. *Nuchal translucency*—measurement first proposed by Benacerraf in 1987 is now found to be an effective marker. It is increased in Trisomy 21 which occurs 1 in 660 live births.
2. Yolk sac measurement have been proposed to be another marker—throughout its existence it has a normal diameter of 3-6 mm with even outline and smooth wall.

3. Single umbilical artery (SUA) and other abnormalities of the cord have been found to be sensitive and specific for many foetal anomalies. Umbilical cord is formed between D13-38 of conception. Two ventral ductal systems namely Vitelline Duct and Allantoic Duct develop also at this embryonic stage which give rise to midgut and hindgut along with umbilical vessel in the latter. Full term umbilical cord is derived from Primary yolk sac, connecting stalk and amnion. Any abnormality in formation thus is associated with structural aberration also in the intestine, abdominal wall and lower limbs. Thus during screening for anomaly it is essential to rule out absence of one umbilical artery, i.e. the entity known as single umbilical artery.

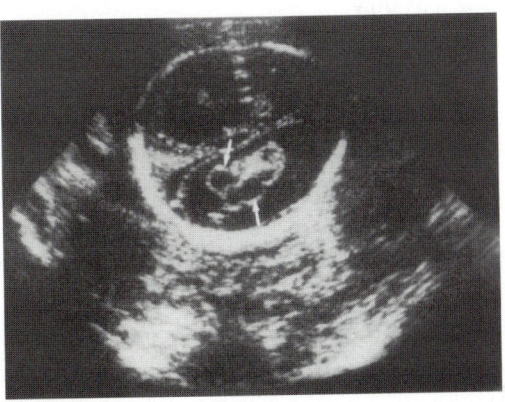

FIGURE 11.7: Choroid plexus cysts—14 weeks

4. Choroid plexus cyst has been reported to be associated with anomalies—however after a large study by Benacerraf, in 1996, (involving 32, 053) it appears that its incidence in 2nd trimester and spontaneous resolution is common. As for occurrence in Trisomy 21, isolated choroid plexus cyst should not be used to increase the patients calculated risk of having a foetus with trisomy 21. However, the risk for trisomy 18 remains. But since spontaneous foetal loss is higher in these chromosomally abnormal pregnancies, the gestational age at detection is important, so is the maternal age.

Congenital Anomaly—Recapitulation

a. Major
b. Minor variety.

Major—those that produce long-term disability and or death.

Minor—compatible with life.

All anomalies are not detectable at birth.

Five major causes of malformation are recognised:

1. Chromosome abnormality—6%
2. Single gene disorder—8% (Approx. 3,000 detected)

3. Teratogenic (environmental)—7% (drug or chemical, infectious agent, radiation, metabolic, e.g. glucose metabolism)
4. Combined or multifactorial—25%
5. Unknown—54%

Incidence of Individual Anomalies

Since majority of severe anomalies are incompatible with growth/life embryonic death occurs early and over 50% first trimester abortus shows chromosomal anomalies. Only **0.5- 0.7%** of live births show major chromosomal anomaly. In order of incidence they are —

Cardiovascular	– 34.4%
Musculoskeletal	– 25.2%
Central nervous system	– 16.8%
Orofacial	– 12.8%
Gastrointestinal	– 3.6%
Abdominal wall defect	– 2.8%
Pulmonary	– 2.5%
Genitourinary	– 1.8%

Single umbilical artery needs special attention during early study since structural and functional abnormality can specifically guide towards major and minor anomalies.

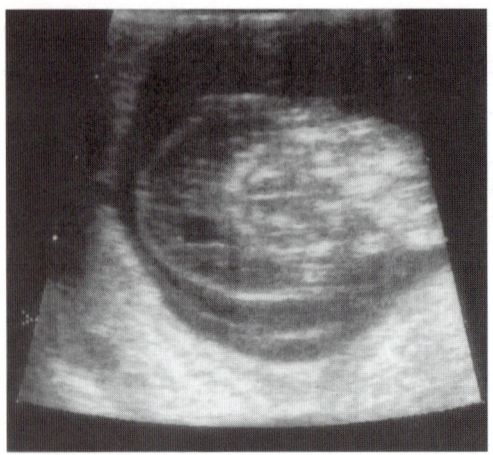

FIGURE 11.8: Nuchal translucency

Early Studies (8–16 weeks) of Cord

Table 11.2

Type of SUA/cord abnormality	Reported associated anomaly
Type 1—Most common variety—98%	CNS, lower genitourinary tract, Acardia
Type 2—Artery present arises from superior mesenteric artery	Sirenomelia, caudal regression, anal agenesis
Type 3—Rare variety	Renal agenesis, limb reduction, hydranencephaly
Type 4—Few cases reported	
Thick cord	DM, macrosomia, hydrops, haemolytic disease
Thin cord	IUGR, IUFD
Varix, angiomyxoma	Unpredictable sudden foetal death
Cyst, pseudocyst aneurysm	Perinatal complication

DETAILED STUDY—GASTROINTESTINAL SYSTEM

Embryology – Primitive gut formation starts at 5th week, intestinal peristalsis starts at 11th week and swallowing starts at 12th weeks. 2-7 ml fluid is swallowed/day at 16th weeks.

Gastrointestinal Anomalies

The stomach is visible to contain fluid by 11 weeks and fluid filled bowel loops often can be seen by 20 weeks. Absence of stomach or enlarged stomach or "double bubble" (30% associated with trisomy 21) signify structural abnormality of different portions of GI tract. Abnormality of liquor volume, commonly seen for GI anomalies, can only be seen in latter part of second trimester, so in early ultrasound for foetal malformation amniotic fluid volume alterations are not usually seen.

Abdominal wall defects—are of 3 major types, gastroschisis, omphalocele, limb—body wall complex (body-stalk anomaly or cyllosomas) minor varieties are also present. Diagnosis by efficient scanning by 16-18 weeks is 97% accurate.

Intra-abdominal anomalies present a particular challenge to the obstetric sonographer since they can arise from a variety of different organs and anatomical sites.

Potential sites of gastrointestinal abnormalities include esophagus, stomach, duodenum, jejuno-ileum and colon, liver, spleen, gallbladder, pancreas and mesentery or peritoneal cavity. Despite the diversity, diagnosis can usually be made after carefully considering the location and sonographic appearance of the abnormality.

Normal Sonographic Appearance

The upper portion of the foetal abdomen is occupied by liver which has a homogeneous echogenicity higher than that of the lungs. At any gestational age, the liver comprises most of the upper abdomen in the foetus.

The most commonly obtained section through the foetal abdomen is the transverse section through the liver at the level of the intrahepatic portion of the umbilical vein. The umbilical vein can be followed from its entrance into the foetal abdomen until the portal sinus. A smaller part of the umbilical vein blood is directed through the ductus venosus can be visualized intrahepatically in the oblique scan.

The gallbladder is normally visualized as an ovoid or pear-shaped fluid-filled structure to the right and inferior to the intrahepatic portion of the umbilical vein. It can be mistaken for the umbilical vein unless the characteristic course of the vein or its intrahepatic branches are visualized.

The foetal stomach becomes visible at the age of 11 menstrual weeks. By 16 weeks, the stomach should be demonstrated in nearly all normal foetuses in the left upper quadrant of the abdomen. It appears as a fluid-filled structure the size and shape of which vary according to the ingestion of amniotic fluid and active peristaltic movements.

Foetal spleen is visualized on a transverse plane just posterior and to the left of the foetal stomach. It appears as a semilunar, hypoechoic structure.

Fluid-filled bowel loops are often seen in the second and third trimester. Distinguishing large bowel from small bowel is possible after 20 menstrual weeks and this distinction becomes more obvious with advancing gestational age. Characteristically, the large bowel appears as a continuous tubular structure located in the periphery of the abdomen and is filled with hypoechoic meconium. The small bowel is located centrally and remains more echogenic in appearance until the late third trimester. The small bowel undergoes peristalsis that can be observed during the third trimester.

Gastrointestinal Obstruction

Most commonly bowel obstruction results in proximal bowel dilatation that is characteristically recognized as one or more tubular or cystic structures within the foetal abdomen. Foetal bowel obstruction may be secondary to a congenital malformation such as intestinal atresia, duplication of the bowel, volvulus, or meconium ileus.

Atresias are the most commonly encountered type of digestive system obstructions.

Esophageal atresia can sometimes be visualized with careful real time scanning. Alternating filling and emptying of a large proximal esophagus can be seen. The presence of swallowing and regurgitation during an ultrasound examination is further presumptive evidence for esophageal atresia. In cases without tracheoesophageal fistula the foetal stomach is not visualized. Esophageal atresia alone would also be expected to cause polyhydramnios. However, demonstration of fluid in the stomach does not necessarily exclude esophageal atresia, since enough fluid may be secreted by the gastric mucosa to make it visible. If the stomach is not visualized, particularly in the presence of polyhydramnios, other congenital anomalies such as diaphragmatic hernia, situs inversus, facial cleft and central nervous system anomalies should also be suspected.

Pyloric atresia is a rare anomaly accounting for approximately 1% of all intestinal atresias. Ultrasound visualization of a dilated, fluid-filled stomach associated with polyhydramnios is highly suggestive of this anomaly.

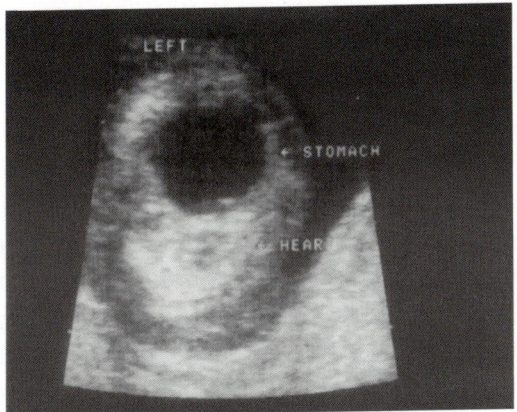

FIGURE 11.9: Dilated foetal stomach

Duodenal atresia has frequently been detected on prenatal sonography. It affects 1 in 5000 pregnancies, and approximately 30% of these are associated with trisomy 21. A characteristic finding is the so-called 'double-bubble' sign, representing the fluid-filled stomach and duodenum. Two round-shaped cystic structures are ultrasonically visualized in the upper abdomen of the affected foetus. The left cyst represents the dilated stomach and the right one is duodenum. Continuity with the stomach should be demonstrated to distinguish a distended duodenum from other cystic masses in the right upper quadrant, such as choledochal cysts and hepatic cysts. Other causes that could produce 'double-bubble' sign include annular pancreas, obstructing bands, volvulus or intestinal duplications.

Normal stomach with prominent incisura angularis should not be mistaken for duodenal atresia. This potential pitfall can be avoided by scanning in a transverse plane.

Intestinal atresia is characterized by several cystic structures in the upper abdomen representing dilated bowel loops. Polyhydramnios is seen less frequently. When dilated small bowel is demonstrated, meconium ileus should be considered as well as jejunoileal atresia and volvulus. Care should be taken to distinguish dilated bowel from hydroureter or other intra-abdominal cystic masses.

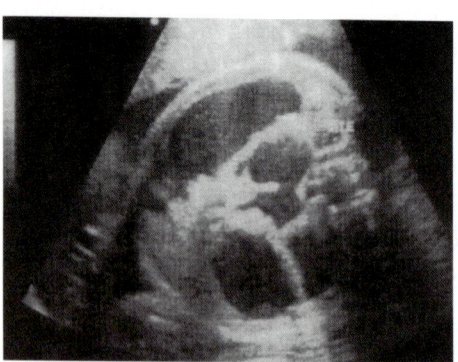

FIGURE 11.10: Dilated bowel loops

More distal obstructions include colonic and anorectal atresias. In distal obstruction there is sufficient length of the proximal bowel for complete resorption of swallowed fluid and polyhydramnios does not occur. Nevertheless, anorectal atresia can sometimes be recognized as dilated colon in the lower abdomen or pelvis. Calcified intraluminal meconium is another possible manifestation of anorectal atresia. Colonic atresia is an isolated anomaly and is extremely rare. Anal atresia is associated with anomalies of other systems (genito-urinary or skeletal) in more than half of cases.

Congenital megacolon (Hirschsprung's disease) is the most common cause of colonic obstruction. It is due to the congenital absence of ganglion cells in the distal intestine. Characteristically, only the rectum and sigmoid colon are involved. Sonogra-phically, severely distended small bowel loops proximally from the site of obstruction and poly-hydramnios can be detected in late pregnancy. However, its manifestation usually occurs later after birth.

Cystic masses arising from the digestive system, excluding dilated bowel are hepatic cysts and tumors, choledochal cyst, enteric duplication cyst, and mesenteric cyst. The prevalence, location and sonographic appearance of cystic malformation can help in making a diagnosis.

Choledochal cyst most frequently results from cystic dilatation of the common bile duct. Other types of choledochal cysts are derived from multiple intrahepatic and extrahepatic cysts, diverticula of the common bile duct and choledochoceles. Chole-dochal cysts are rare and can be identified as a

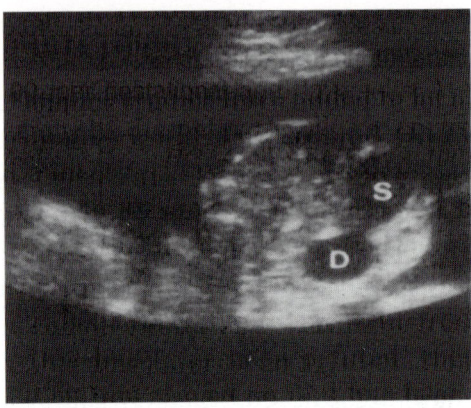

FIGURE 11.11: "Double bubble" sign

simple cystic mass in the upper abdomen or right upper quadrant.

Enteric duplication cysts may occur at any level along the gastrointestinal tract. The stomach is involved less frequently than other regions. On prenatal sonography, duplication cysts are seen as cystic intra-abdominal masses that should be distinguished from mesenteric or omental cysts, urachal cyst, ovarian cyst or hepatic cyst.

The sonographic findings of mesenteric, omental and retroperitoneal cysts are variable. They can be unilocular or multiseptate and of various sizes. Usually sonolucent, they may appear solid when hemorrhagic. They are usually located in mid abdomen. Mesenteric and omental cysts are characteristically mobile.

Normal Anatomy and Malformations of Foetal Abdominal Wall

Abdominal wall defects occur early in embryological development. Routine views of the anterior abdominal wall and umbilical cord insertion site are recommended. A false-positive diagnosis of abdominal wall defect is possible between 6 and 12 weeks when the rapidly elongating midgut normally herniates into the base of the body stalk. Because of this embryologic process, a reliable diagnosis of gastroschisis or omphalocele may not be possible before 12 weeks.

Omphalocele

This is defined as a herniation of variable amount of abdominal viscera into the base of the umbilical cord. It results from a failure of the intestine to return to the abdomen or from a failure of four embryonic disc folds to fuse into the primitive pleuroperitoneal cavity. The result of fusion failure is a midline abdominal wall defect. The viscera are covered with a membranous sac of peritoneum and amnion. The umbilical cord inserts into the sac with it vessels spreading within the sac wall. The herniated sac contains, according to the degree of the defect, the intestines, liver, stomach and spleen. If the sac ruptures prenatally, an omphalocele could be mistaken for gastroschisis. Regardless of the size of the defect in the foetal skin, the underlying rectus muscles are intact.

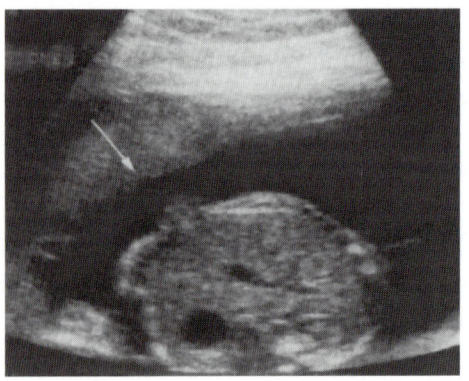

FIGURE 11.12: Omphalocele

Sonographically, omphalocele may demonstrate a variable appearance depending on the size of the abdominal wall defect, type of eviscerated organs, presence of ascites and associated anomalies. The primary diagnostic features of omphalocele is the central location of the abdominal wall defect at the base of the umbilical cord insertion site. The presence of a limiting membrane is another essential feature of omphalocele.

Chromosome abnormalities have been reported in 10-40% of neonates with omphalocele, mostly trisomies 18 and 13. In view of this, the prenatal work-up should include a complete ultrasound evaluation of the affected foetus.

Gastroschisis

This is an abdominal wall defect mainly located in the right paraumbilical region. The defect involves all layers of the abdominal wall and is usually 2-5 cm in size. It has been suggested that gastroschisis results from abnormal involution of the right umbilical vein or from the disruption of the omphalomesenteric artery. Gastroschisis is sporadic, and no genetic association or recurrence risks have been described. The ultrasonic finding of bowel loops floating in the amniotic fluid outside the foetal abdomen is characteristic. As the defect is located paraumbilically, the umbilical cord is inserted normally.

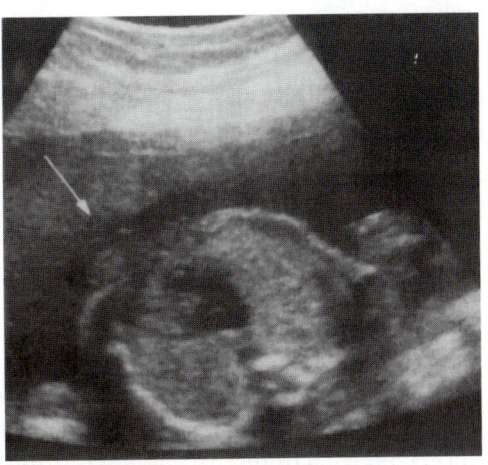

FIGURE 11.13: Gastroschisis

Congenital Diaphragmatic Hernia

Ultrasound diagnosis of diaphragmatic hernia is based upon three characteristic signs: Polyhydramnios, mediastinal shift and inability to visualize stomach in its normal place in the upper abdomen. As most hernias contain the small bowel, bowel loops can be seen in the thoracic cavity. The fluid-filled stomach and small bowel contrast to the more echogenic foetal lung especially in the left-sided hernias.

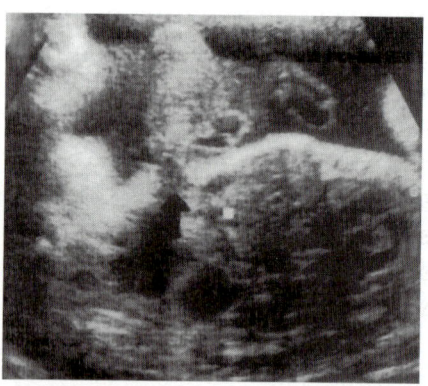

FIGURE 11.14: Gastroschisis

Cloacal and Bladder Extrophy

These share a common embryologic origin in abnormal cloacal development – Bladder extrophy is characterized by a defect in the lower abdominal wall and anterior wall of the urinary bladder.

Cloacal extrophy results in extrophy of the bladder, in which there are two hemibladders separated by intestinal mucosa. Other malformations include abdominal and pelvic defects, anorectal atresia and spinal abnormalities.

GENITOURINARY SYSTEM

Embryology from 6th week mesonephric (Wolfian) duct forms from urogenital sinus. An out pouching from it gives rise to ureteric bud from which down 15 generations the ureter, renal pelvis, calyx, and collecting tubule formation starts. Nephrons form by 10 weeks and urine production commences at 11 weeks thus making the bladder visible by 12 weeks. However, this urine formation does not contribute to amniotic fluid volume till 16 weeks. So nonvisualization of urinary bladder around 12-14 weeks on repeated study should hint towards some abnormality in urine production and detailed study of kidneys performed.

Edith L Potter : "The more complicated an organ in its development the more subject it is to mal-development and in this respect the kidney outranks most other organs" (Table 11.3).

CARDIOVASCULAR SYSTEM

Heart is the first organ to start functioning at 5 weeks pulsating at 110 beats/min. The rate goes

Table 11.3: Varieties of kidney anomaly

Disease	Ultrasound Features
Potter Type I (Autosomal recessive)	Bilaterally enlarged hyperechoic kidney
Potter Type II (Multicystic/Dysplastic)	
(A)	Segmental involvement in normal or enlarged kidney
(B)	Rudimentary kidney with small cyst
Potter Type III (Autosomal dominant)	Manifests in 3rd and 5th decades
Potter Type IV (Cystic disease due to urethral obstruction)	Fluid filled urinary tract

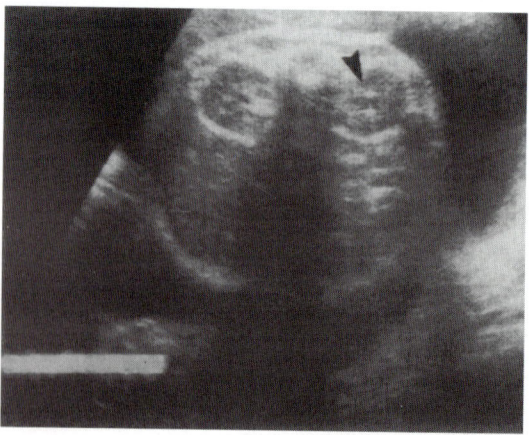

FIGURE 11.15: Dilated ureter at renal pelvis

on rising till 9 weeks to reach 175/min then vagal innervation proceeds and rate of cardiac contraction settles between 150-160/min. Four chamber view is essential for diagnosis of anomaly. Great vessel at exit can be seen and with CD detailed Cardiac Study is possible by 15 weeks. However, for diagnostic purposes cardiac study can be complete around 18th week when the antero-posterior diameter becomes 1.5 cm. The normal cardiac diameter around this time is approximately 13% of CRL.

Normal Anatomy and Malformation of the Foetal Cardiovascular System

The Four Chamber View

Approximately 70-80% of congenital heart abnormalities can be excluded from a normal four chamber view.

On ultrasound the four chamber view is presented as follows.

- The heart fills approximately one-third of the foetal thorax;
- The right and left atria are approximately equal in size;
- The right and left ventricular cavities are more or less equal in size at the level of the valves;
- The right ventricle is closest to the sternum, the left atrium closest to the spine.
- Mitral and tricuspid valves open with each cardiac cycle;

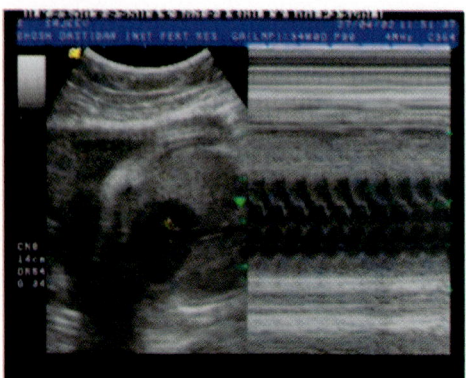

FIGURE 11.16: Foetal echocardiography

- Ventricular walls and interventricular septum are more or less equal in thickness;
- The tricuspid valve inserts lower than the mitral valve;
- The right ventricular apex has a 'triangular' shape due to increased trabeculations and the moderator band;
- The foramen ovale flap is seen with movement into the left atrium;
- The pulmonary veins insert into the left atrium— seen on either side of the spinal crest; and
- The ventricular septum appears intact.

Left Heart Connections

From the four chamber position cranial angulation of the transducer produces the 'fifth chamber view'

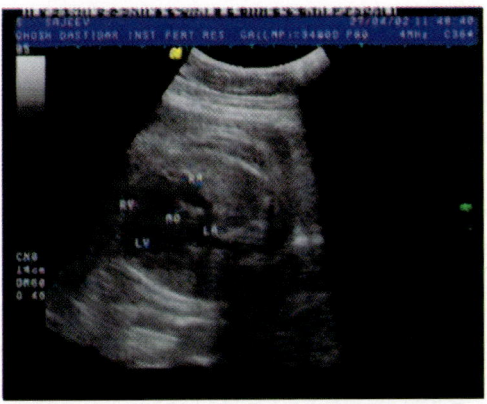

FIGURE 11.17: Five chamber view of foetal heart

or the four-chamber aortic root view. Turning the transducer lengthwise will produce a left ventricular long axis view. Continuity between the anterior wall of the aorta and interventricular septum, and the posterior wall of the aorta and anterior mitral valves leaflet should be identified. Still turning the transducer longitudinally shows the aortic arch with innominate, carotid and subclavian arteries to the head and neck. The ascending aorta lies to the right of the main pulmonary artery and angles out to the right.

Right Heart Connections

The pulmonary artery is closer to the chest wall and runs straight towards the spine. Focussing the transducer along the length of the right ventricular outflow tract shows the pulmonary valve. Scanning the base of the heart lengthwise brings the inferior and superior vena caval connections into view. Further angulation in a horizontal direction visualizes the main pulmonary artery, right and left pulmonary arteries and or the ductus arteriosus. A parasternal short axis view shows both ventricles, the right rather elongated and the left seen as a circle, 'sitting' on the diaphragm.

RESPIRATORY SYSTEM

The upper respiratory system can be partially seen by ultrasound. Portions of the pharynx and hypopharynx are commonly visible because of the presence of fluid. Details of laryngeal anatomy are not particularly evident but the larynx itself can be easily recognized as a superior constriction of the tracheal fluid column. The trachea can be easily visualized due to the fact that it is consistently filled with fluid. Mainstream bronchi are usually invisible.

The foetal chest can be easily recognized by using the foetal heart as a landmark. Respiratory movements are also visible in early second trimester.

The lung tissue can be seen from the late first trimester onward. The structures that surround it include ribs, heart and liver. Sonography routinely visualizes the foetal lungs by the mid-second trimester. They appear as two moderately and homogeneously echogenic areas on either side of the heart. On longitudinal section the diaphragm can be recognized between the lungs and the liver as a relatively transonic line moving during respiratory excursions. Lung echogenicity increases after 35-36 weeks, approaching that of the liver. It has been suggested that foetal pulmonic maturity has been achieved when lung echogenicity is equal to, or greater than liver echogenicity.

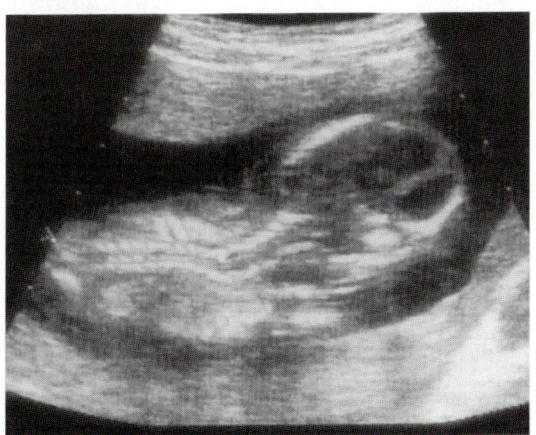

FIGURE 11.18: Deformed spine, ribs—asphyxiating thoracic dysplasia

Impaired maturation of foetal lungs frequently results in postnatal respiratory distress or death. Derangements of the intrauterine environment, thorax, (Fig. 11.18) or extrathoracic organ systems profoundly affect the prenatal development of the lungs. Pulmonary hypoplasia detected prenatally usually occurs in prolonged and severe oligohyd-ramnios due to poor bathing of pulmonary tissue or primary thoracic abnormalities. In the case of an abnormal thoracic mass or pleural fluid collec-tion, evaluation of the size may assist in prediction of associated pulmonary hypoplasia. The severity of pulmonary hypoplasia depends upon the gesta-tional age of onset, duration of the inciting condi-tions and severity of the insult. The foetal thorax normally grows at a regular rate from 16 to 40 weeks.

Hydrothorax is abnormal foetal pleural fluid col-lection developed from various etiologies. Excluding hydrops, the most common cause of fluid accumu-lation in the foetal thorax is chylothorax. Chylo-thorax is particularly likely when the pleural effusion is unilateral. The right side is affected more often than the left, and males twice as often as females. Congenital chylothorax probably results from a malformation of the foetal thoracic duct. The specific diagnosis is made postnatally, because prior to oral milk feeding the fluid appears clear.

Hydrothorax produces an anechoic space located on the periphery of the thoracic cavity. Anechoic pleural fluid collection displaces the lungs away from the chest wall and compresses the lungs which might result in improper growth. The partially collapsed lungs usually retain their normal shape.

Cystic adenomatoid malformation of the lung (CAML) is a lung hamartoma with overgrowth of the mesenchymal elements. Type I contains one or several large cysts ranging from 2 to 10 cm in diameter, and small cysts along the periphery of the hemithorax. These cysts can involve the entire lobe. Type II has multiple small cysts measuring less than 1 cm in diameter. On ultrasound scan, type II creates a mass with numerous small cysts. Type III creates a large solid mass involving the entire lobe. It produces a homogeneous echogenic mass without individual cysts. It has been associated with a number of genetic disorders or also seen isolated. Many of these cases have been reported to resolute at later study.

MUSCULOSKELETAL ANOMALY

One hundred twenty five skeletal dysplasias have till now been described, nine perinatal deaths out of every thousand is due to skeletal dysplasia. Many of these cases have shown genetic mutation and have an abnormality of : Fibroblast growth factor receptor abnormality (FGFRA).

Evaluation of the Long Bones

Long bone evaluation includes the assessment of their length, shape and degree of mineralization. By comparing the different bone segments, the type of limb shortening can be established.

In evaluating the shape of a long bone, the degree of its curvature and the possibility of fractures should be considered. Excessive bowing ('campomelia') is characteristic of campomelic dysplasia and osteogenesis imperfecta; fractures are typical of osteogenesis imperfecta and hypophosphatasia.

Finally the degree of mineralization of long bones should be assessed by examining the echogenicity of the bone and its acoustic shadow.

Evaluation of the foetal extremities should include also the hands and feet, looking for polydactyly or syndactyly, and extreme postural deformities, such as those seen in diastrophic dysplasia. Cloverleaf skull deformity is typical of thanatophoric dwarphism. Bone demineralization, typical of congenital hypophosphatasia and osteogenesis imperfecta, produces an impressive ultrasonic visualization of intracranial structures. Furthermore the skull is very thin and can be easily deformed by a slight compression of the ultrasound probe. Evaluation of the orbits allows the recognition of hypo and hypertelorism. By observing the foetal profile anomalies such as frontal bossing, depressed nasal bridge, cleft palate and micrognathia can be recognized.

Skeletal Deformities of the Thorax

Several skeletal dysplasias are associated with hypoplastic thorax (achondrogenesis, thanato-

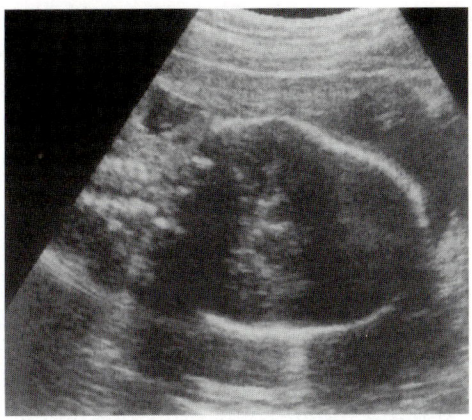

FIGURE 11.19: Deformed skull

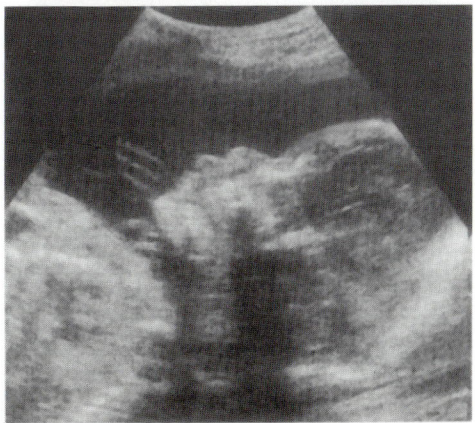

FIGURE 11.20: Depressed nasal bridge

phoric dwarphism, asphyxiating thoracic dysplasia, etc), Chest restriction may lead to pulmonary hypoplasia, a frequent cause of death in these conditions. Thoracic dimensions can be evaluated by measuring the thoracic circumference at the level of the heart.

Ultrasonic Findings Typical for Specific Dysplasias

Cloverleaf skull (thanatophoric dysplasia)
Hitch-hiker thumbs (diastrophic dysplasia)
Spine demineralization (achondrogenesis)
Hypoplastic scapulae (campomelic dysplasia)
Acromesomelia (chondroectodermal dysplasia)

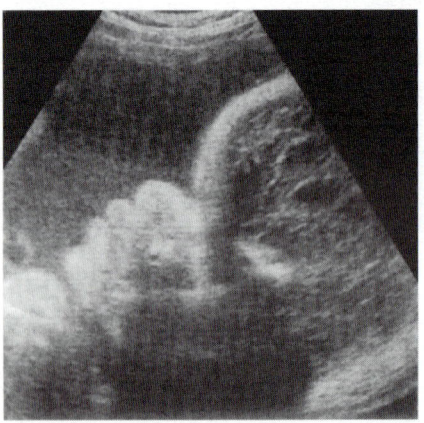

FIGURE 11.21: Frontal 'bossing'

Neural Tube Defects (NTD) – seen 1 in 500 births has been classified to be primary cranial or primary spinal, skeletal anomaly.

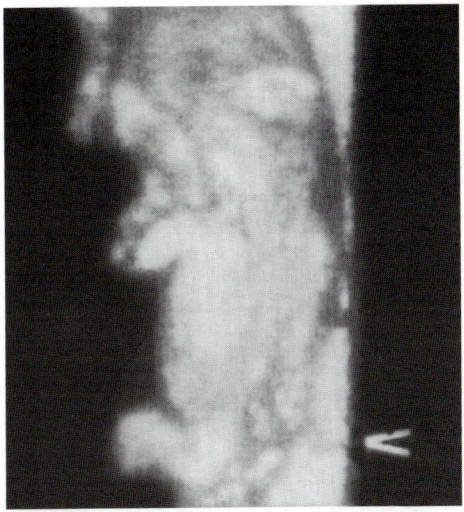

FIGURE 11.22: 3D view—Meningomyelocele

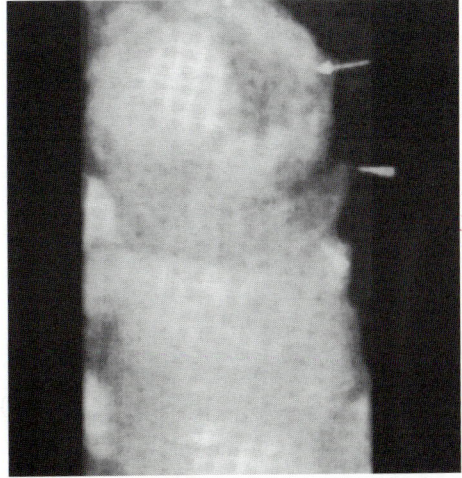

FIGURE 11.23: Vault deformity—3D view

Absence of cranial vault gives rise to anencephaly seen on ultrasound from 12th week as 'Toad face" or "Mickey mouse appearance". Spinal defects may be closed or open. On ultrasound "splaying' of vertebra or a mass like meningomyelocele seen.

Amniotic bands and sheets seen within the amniotic cavity attach to foetal parts and may result in minor or major deformities.

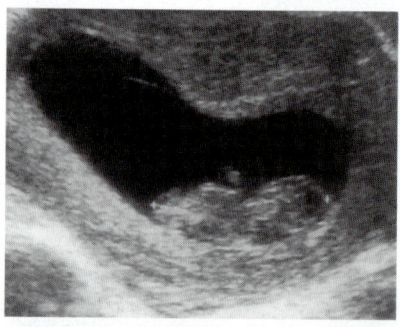

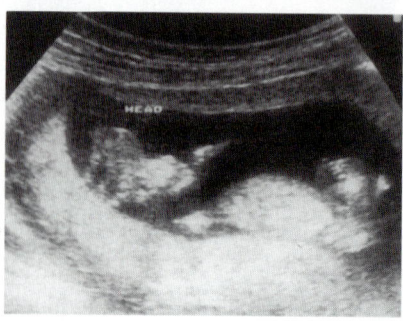

FIGURE 11.24: Compare normal vault with anencephaly

Concluding Remarks

Routine foetal anomaly study had been advocated at 18-20 weeks for a very long time. However, as workers all over the world had began to realize that it is actually possible to see the anatomy and physiology of sonoembryology from a very early period and since most of the organogenesis is complete and functional by 14 weeks the last being the brain formation - 18 weeks, it appears prudent to advocate early ultrasound screening for foetal malformation around 16 weeks.

The markers however, would lead one to believe that early study can also be complete by 13-14 weeks.

Chapter 12
Safety

The question of bio-effects of any diagnostic technique remains foremost in the minds of all workers involved in this aspect of medical science. The effect of the used technology on the patient and health worker is of equal importance. Since, ultrasound has found an exceptionally prominent place in obstetrics, its effect on the unborn life, i.e. foetus is also of great significance.

Though reports of increase in frequency of Sister Chromatid Exchanges (SCE) in human lymphocyte cells, in response to in vitro exposure to pulsed ultrasound at diagnostic levels has been reported, similar follow-up studies in animal experiments upto 20 generations following initial insonation has not shown any adverse effect. But since cells of culture system is different from the intact patient and the foetus is well guarded within maternal tissue, experimental results should be correlated to clinical condition with great caution.

Though no adverse effect has been confirmed it is wise to assume that a potential risk might exist and precaution must be taken to minimize this hypothetical risk. Theoretically the mechanism by which ultrasound could adversely affect the explored tissue, as has been seen in its surgical and therapeutical uses, is by—(1) heating effect, (2) mechanical effect. However, the effects thus reported have been induced by ultrasound at intensity levels above those used for diagnostic purposes.

No genetic effect has also been proved. Epidemiological studies have been undertaken to relate human exposure to diagnostic ultrasound and disease. Such studies, concerned with factors that influence pattern of occurance of disease, in this case, searching relation of in utero ultrasound exposure and childhood—maldevelopment, malignancy, neurological deficit, delayed speech development, low birth weight and delayed growth could not correlate such relation in large work up undertaken till date. However, pulsed Doppler is not recommended in the study of first few weeks of gestation.

Continuous Doppler ultrasound monitoring for prolonged period during labour associated with increase in erythrocyte fragility must be viewed with concern. Thus it has been postulated that careful and prudent use of diagnostic ultrasound is advisable in situations were not doing the ultrasound study would be more harmful to the patient. The bio-effects committee of American Institute of Ultrasound in Medicine has a similar opinion.

Many research groups like the National Council on Radiation Protection (NCRP) and Measurements, The Institute of Physical Sciences in Medicine, World Federation of Ultrasound in Medicine and Biology, International Society of Ultrasound in Obstetrics and Gynaecology, National Electrical manufacturers' Association (USA) are giving the safety factor serious thought.

Table 12.1

Diagnostic ultrasound	Approximate intensity range (SATA*) in mw/cm
1) Perivascular Doppler	500 - 50
2) Others	50 - 1

* SATA - Spatial average, temporal average.

Salutation to the Giants on whose Shoulders we Rest

1. **Vesalius (1543):** For giving us the true concept of pelvic anatomy in "De Humani Corporis Fabrica".

2. **Christian Doppler (1853):** Explanation of "The red shift in light from stars" published in his paper "On the coloured light of double stars and certain other stars of the heavens" which has relevance to present day medical ultrasound.

3. **Professor William J. Fry (1939-45):** Studied piezoelectric transducers at the Naval Research Laboratory in Washington DC during World War II and installed a high intensity focused system. This was used to produce trackless surgical lesions in brain for psychological and neurological disorders and also for destruction of pituitary gland in patients thought to have hormone dependant cancer.

4. **J. J. Wild, Reid J. M. Howry DH and Bliss Wr. (1952):** Development of water bath coupling to study soft tissue.

5. **Editor I, Hertz CH (1954):** Ultrasonographic recording of cardiac movements made possible.

6. **S. Satomura (1957):** Based on "Doppler Shift" discovered that blood flow studies could be done studying shift in frequency of back-scattered ultrasound.

7. **Ian Donald, Mac Vicar and Brown (1959):** Studies on pregnant uterus made possible.

8. **George Kossof (1962):** Developed transducers to "see' foetal anatomy.

9. **PNT Wells (1966):** Developed the articulated arm static scanner.

10. **Stuart Campbell (1969):** Developed definite parameters for foetal study.

11. **George Kossof (1969):** Now he modified old machines for time lapse photography and hence developed technology of 'grey scale'.

12. **J. M. Griffith and Henry WL (1974):** Made real time echo-cardiography possible.

13. **FE Barber, DW Baker (1974):** Developed the duplex scanner.

14. **C. Kasai, K Namekawa, A. Koyano (1958):** Based on Doppler principle, showed that real time 2D imaging of blood flow is possible.

15. To all the other silent workers who toiled through the last 25 years to lay the path on which we now tread.

Recent Additions to Ultrasound Technology

1. Two dimensional color flow imaging.
2. Endovaginal scanning - has added "eyes" to our fingertips.
3. Extracorporeal shockwave lithotripsy.
4. Ultrasonic hyperthermia for treatment of cancer.
5. Intraluminal transducers.
6. Contrast agents for ultrasound.
7. Three dimensional imaging in ultrasound - even helps people not specialized in imaging understand images.
8. Volume flow rate measurements by Pulsed Doppler.

Possible Future Development

1. Development of targeted contrast agents which might replace much of nuclear medicine.
2. With proliferation of ultrasound imaging information, it will essentially be integrated in "Image Management and Communications Systems" (IMACS).
3. Pocket-sized imaging instruments—however this will enhance risk of diagnostic errors.
4. To fully utilize the 3-D technology, interpretation of anatomical appearances viewed from a "mobile point that can be navigated anywhere within the scanned volume combined with time

as the fourth dimension" will have to be mastered—4D.

5. "Simulated intervention" - much in the same manner in which aeroplane pilots are trained, surgeons will be able to plan approaches.

6. Real time colour flow imaging of gynaecological physiology, pathology and that of feto-maternal haemodynamics will be standardized.

There is a galaxy of opportunities waiting to be explored and we strongly believe that the next 25 years will be as exciting as the past, if not more.

Bibliography

1. Campbell S, Wilkin D. Ultrasonic measurement of fetal abdomen circumference in the estimation of fetal weight. *Br J Obstet Gynaecol* **82**: 689-97, 1975.
2. Campbell S. The prediction of fetal maturity by ultrasonic measurement of the biparietal diameter. *J Obstet Gynaecol Br Commonw* **76**: 605-09, 1969.
3. Campbell S, Diaz-Recasens J, Griffin DR, Cohen-Overbeek TE, Pearce JM, Willson K, Teague MJ. New Doppler technique for assessing utero-placental blood flow. *Lancet*, **1**: 675-77, 1983.
4. Campbell S, Warsof SL, Little D, Cooper DJ. Routine ultrasound screening for the prediction of gestational age. *Obstet Gynecol* **65**: 613-20, 1985.
5. Cousins L. Congenital anomalies among infants of diabetic mothers: Etiology, prevention, diagnosis. *Am J Obstet Gynecol* **147:** 333-38
6. Ghosh Dastidar Kakoli. Chapter on Role of Transvaginal Colour Doppler in Gynaecology – in Endosonography in Obsterics & Gynaecology, Published by – Rotunda Medical Technologies Pvt. Ltd. India.
7. Ghosh Dastidar Kakoli. Interventional Transvaginal Sonography – Indian Journal of Medical Ultrasound, Vol. 12, No. 3&4, P 6-13, 1995.
8. Ghosh Dastidar Kakoli. Studies by Doppler Ultrasound for comparison of uterine blood flow parameters in normo-ovulatory and dysovulatory (PCO) subjects – Journal of Obst. & Gyn. of India, **51(1):** 89-91, 2001.
9. Ghosh Dastidar Kakoli, Ghosh Dastidar Sudarsan. Further Studies on Earliest Ultrasound Findings of Implantation – Journal of Assisted Reproduction & Genetics, **14(5):** 1997

10. Ghosh Dastidar Kakoli, Ghosh Dastidar Sudarsan, Doppler studies on vascularity of implanting trophoblast following embryo transfer : Ultra. Obstet. Gynecol., Vol 12, supplement 1 (abstract), 86, 1998.

11. Ghosh Dastidar Kakoli, Ghosh Dastidar Sudarsan, Roy Chowdhury NN. Proceedings of the International Conference on Advances in Reproductive Medicine – (ICARM'97). Bhadra Printer, 1997.

12. Ghosh Dastidar Kakoli, Ghosh Dastidar Sudarsan: Ultrasound Studies on Implantation of Embroys in ART Cycles – The Journal of Obstetrics & Gynaecology of India, Vo. 48, No.1, Feb. '98, P-64-66, ISSN-0971-9202.

13. Ghosh Dastidar Sudarsan, Ghosh Dastidar Kakoli : Comparison of intraovarian stromal vascular Doppler characteristics in PCO patients before & after treatment – Proceedings of the 10th World Congress of In Vitro Fertilization & Assisted Reproduction, Vancouver (Canada), May 24-28, 1997, Monduzzi Editore.

14. Ghosh Dastidar Sudarsan, Ghosh Dastidar Kakoli : Earliest Ultrasound Finding of Implantation – Journal of Assisted Reproduction & Genetics, Vol. 14, No.3, 1997.

15. Ghosh Dastidar Sudarsan, S Panja, Ghosh DD, Dastidar Ghosh Kakoli: Transvaginal Sonography prior to Laparoscopic examination helps to diagnose deep ovarian Endometrioma – Journal of Obstetrics and Gynaecology of India – Vol. 46, No.2, April '96.

16. Gosling RG, King DH. *Ultrasound angiology – In:* Harcus AW, Adamson J (Eds). Arteries and Veins. Edinburgh: Churchill Livingstone.

17. Hadlock FP, Harrist RB, Sharma RS. Estimation of fetal weight with the use of head, body and femur measurements. *Am J Obstet Gynecol* **151**, 333-37, 1985.

18. Kaback MM in Rodeck CH, Nicolaides KM (Eds). The utility of prenatal Diagnosis –Perinatal Diagnosis, N. Y. John Wiley. 1984.

19. L Engmann, P Sladkevicius, R Agarwal, J Bekin, S Campbell, SL Tan : The pattern of changes in ovarian

stromal and uterine artery blood flow velocities during in vitro fertilization treatment and its relationship with outcomes of the cycle. *Ultra Obstet Gynaecol* **13**: 26-33.

20. Morrison I. Perinatal Mortality: Basic Considerations –Semin Perinatal, **9**: 144-50, 1985.

21. Moulik D, Nanda NC, Saini VD. Fetal Doppler echocardiography: Methods and characterization of normal and abnormal haemodynamics. *Am J Cardiol* **53**: 572, 1984.

22. Moulik D, Saini VD, Nanda NC, Resinzweig MS. Doppler evaluation of fetal haemodynamies. *Ultrasound Med Biol*,**8**: 705, 1982.

23. Polson DW *et al.* Polycystic Ovaries – a common finding in normal women. *Lancet*, **1**: 870-72.

24. Poretsky L, Piper B: Insulin resistance, hypersecretion of LH and a dual defect hypothesis for the pathogenesis of polycystic ovary syndrome. *Obstet Gynecol* **84**: 613-21, 1994.

25. Seang Lin Tan Clinical applications of Doppler and three dimensional ultrasound in assisted reproductive technology. *Ultra Obstet Gynaecol* **13**: 157-160.

26. W Schuth, U Karele, C Wilhelm, S Reisch. Parent's needs after ultrasound diagnosis of a fetal malformation: An empirical deficit analysis. *Ultrasound Obstet Gynaecol* **4**: 124-29, 1995.

27. Wladimiroff JW, *et al.* Cerebral and umbilical arterial blood flow velocity waveform in normal and growth retarded pregnancies. *Obstet Gynaecol* **69**: 705-09, 1987.

Index